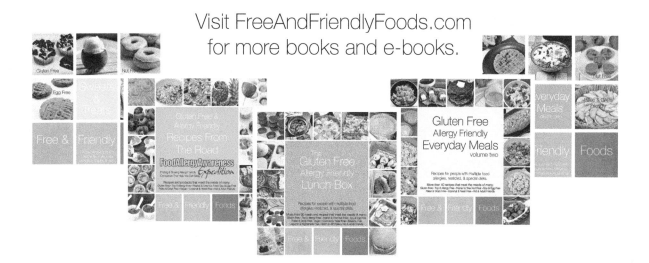
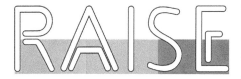

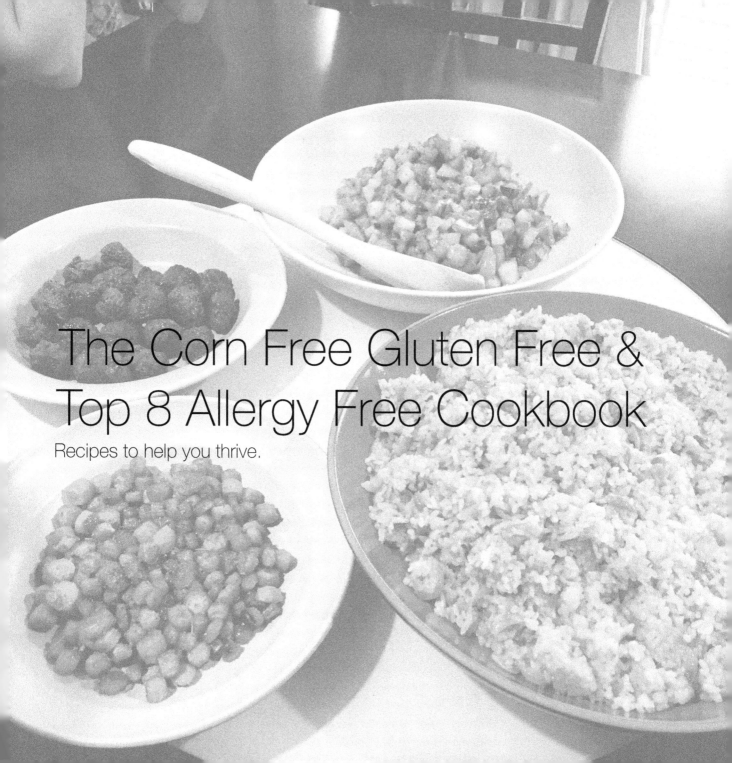

The Corn Free Gluten Free & Top 8 Allergy Free Cookbook

Recipes to help you thrive.

Dedicated to Doug and Dean.

Special thanks to our near and dear corn free friends:
Colleen, Laura, and Mena.

Written and Photographed by
Free & Friendly Foods, LLC
© Copyright 2018

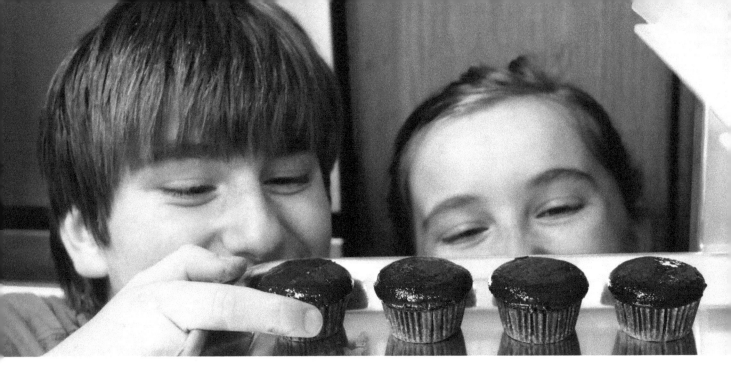

Designed, Edited, Produced, Directed, and Styled by the Free & Friendly Foods Team.

US Library of Congress cataloging-in-publication data has been applied for.

Disclaimer

The recipes in this book are not medical advice. Please consult with your doctor or allergist if necessary before trying any of these items. If you feel you are having a medical emergency, seek help and dial 9-1-1.

Need Help?

We are always happy to help people with any questions they may have. If you're new to the food allergy community, or need help with a recipe, don't hesitate to reach out. Find us online at freeandfriendlyfoods.com. We also have a blog at foodandlego.com.

ISBN 978-1-945374-11-1
© Copyright 2018

Contents

The Helpful & Popular Chart

Here are the recipes, in order of appearance, with notes on their allergy status. Happy cooking & baking!

Recipe	Pg.	Freeze Well	GF	Top 8	CF	Leg Free	Ses Free	Nts Free	CSF	Veg	LH	Paleo	AIP
Oat Milk	32	✓	✓	✓	✓	✓	✓	✓	✓	✓	✓	✗	✗
Tiger Nut Milk	32	✓	✓	✓	✓	✓	✓	✓	✓	✓	✓	✓	✓
Grape Slushie	35	✓	✓	✓	✓	✓	✓	✓	✓	✓	✓	✓	✓
Maple Slushie	36	✓	✓	✓	✓	✓	✓	✓	✓	✓	✓	✓	✓
Avocado Cream Sauce	39	✗	✓	✓	✓	✓	✓	✓	✓	✓	✓	✓	✓
Ketchup	40	✗	✓	✓	✓	✓	✓	✓	✓	✓	✗	✓	✗
Pesto	42	✓	✓	✓	✓	✓	✓	✓	✓	✓	✓	✓	✳
BBQ Sauce	43	✗	✓	✓	✓	✓	✓	✗	✗	✓	✗	✗	✗
Vanilla Ice Cream	46	✓	✓	✓	✓	✓	✓	✓	✓	✓	✓	✓	✳
Chocolate Ice Cream	49	✓	✓	✓	✓	✓	✓	✗	✗	✓	✗	✗	✗
Sunflower Chocolate Chip Cookies	50	✓	✓	✓	✓	✓	✓	✓	✓	✓	✳	✓	✗
Salted Oat Cookie Loaf	53	✓	✓	✓	✓	✓	✓	✓	✓	✓	✓	✗	✗
Jam Crumble	58	✗	✓	✓	✓	✓	✓	✓	✓	✓	✗	✓	✗
Grain Free Waffle	62	✓	✓	✓	✓	✓	✓	✓	✓	✓	✗	✓	✓
Green Shake Smoothie	65	✓	✓	✓	✓	✓	✓	✓	✓	✓	✓	✓	✓

GF = Gluten Free   Top 8 = Free From Wheat, Dairy, Eggs, Soy, Peanuts, Tree Nuts & Coconut, Fish, Shellfish   CF = Corn Free

Leg Free = Legume Free   Ses Free = Sesame Free   Nts Free = Nightshade Free   CSF = Cane Sugar Free

Veg = Vegan   LH = Low Histamine   AIP = Autoimmune Protocol

✓ Good to Go   ✗ No Go   ✳ ✳ Batter/Raw Materials Only   ✳ Modifications Needed

Recipe	Pg.	Freeze Well	GF	Top 8	CF	Leg Free	Ses Free	Nts Free	CSF	Veg	LH	Paleo	AIP
Cinnamon Oat Pancakes	66	✳✳	✓	✓	✓	✓	✓	✗	✓	✓	✗	✗	✗
Bacon Bison Meatballs	69	✓	✓	✓	✓	✓	✓	✓	✓	✗	✗	✓	✓
Cinnamon Pancakes	70	✳✳	✓	✓	✓	✓	✓	✗	✓	✓	✗	✓	✓
Bread	77	✗	✓	✓	✓	✓	✓	✓	✓	✓	✗	✓	✗
Garlic Knots	78	✗	✓	✓	✓	✓	✓	✓	✓	✓	✗	✓	✗
Garlic Meatballs	81	✓	✓	✓	✓	✓	✓	✓	✓	✗	✗	✓	✓
Mini Bison Pockets	82	✓	✓	✓	✓	✓	✓	✓	✓	✗	✓	✗	✗
Bison Dumpling Soup	85	✗	✓	✓	✓	✓	✓	✓	✓	✗	✓	✳	✳
Pulled BBQ Bison	86	✓	✓	✓	✓	✓	✓	✗	✓	✗	✳	✓	✗
Veggie Soup	89	✗	✓	✓	✓	✓	✓	✗	✓	✓	✓	✗	✗
Veggie Bison Meatballs	90	✓	✓	✓	✓	✓	✓	✓	✓	✗	✓	✓	✓
Fried Cauliflower	93	✗	✓	✓	✓	✓	✓	✗	✓	✓	✗	✗	✗
Honey Mustard Bacon & Potatoes	94	✗	✓	✓	✓	✓	✓	✗	✓	✗	✗	✗	✗
Tacos	97	✗	✓	✓	✓	✓	✓	✓	✓	✗	✳	✳	✳
Bacon Bomb Potatoes	98	✗	✓	✓	✓	✓	✓	✗	✓	✓	✓	✗	✗

GF = Gluten Free   Top 8 = Free From Wheat, Dairy, Eggs, Soy, Peanuts, Tree Nuts & Coconut, Fish, Shellfish   CF = Corn Free

Leg Free = Legume Free   Ses Free = Sesame Free   Nts Free = Nightshade Free   CSF = Cane Sugar Free

Veg = Vegan   LH = Low Histamine   AIP = Autoimmune Protocol

✓ Good to Go   ✗ No Go   ✳ ✳ Batter/Raw Materials Only   ✳ Modifications Needed

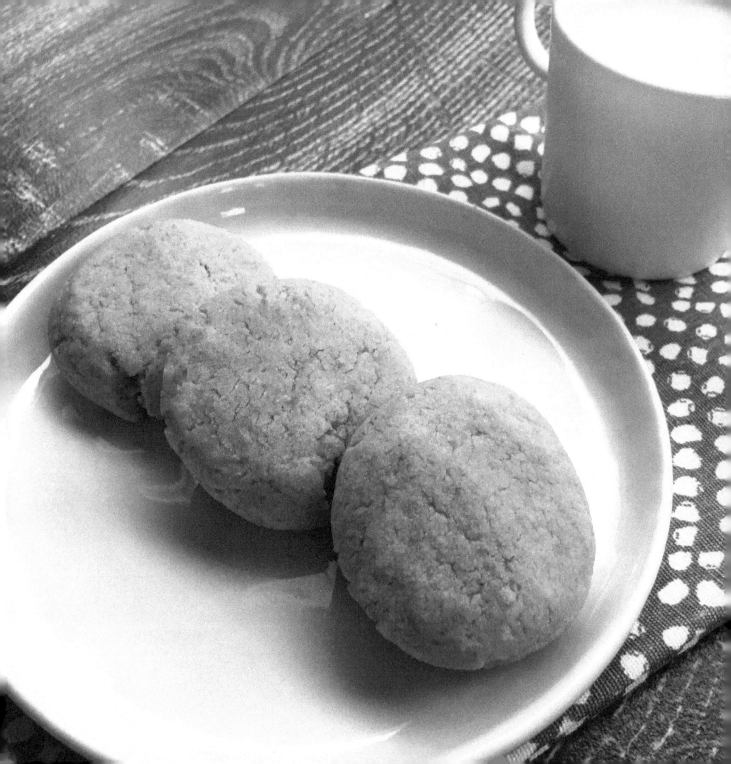

Introduction

Hello Everyone! No matter why you're here, we're so glad you found this book, and we hope it brings joy to your kitchen. There are three major things to consider when you're diagnosed with a corn allergy: Air, Food, and Water. You can't live without them, and they all contain corn. Be sure you're keeping a very detailed food journal that tracks every tiny symptom along with where you've been, what you've consumed, how you've slept, and restroom patterns. I suggest a digital journal, as it's much easier to search through later. Back to those three items. Depending on the severity of your corn allergy, you may only need to avoid ingesting actual corn (cob, starch, meal, etc.). Others may not be able to have corn or its derivatives (over 200 including xanthan gum). When it comes to water, most of you will be fine with tap water. Others will require a Big Berkey (ceramic filters) or water from Summit Spring/Tourmaline Spring. When it comes to air, 90% of you will be just fine. The rest us may require an I Can Breathe mask, or a 3M Full Face Respirator, as ethanol (corn) is in most gasoline. However, don't let any of this scare you off. It's a really hard diagnosis to cope with, but once you get the hang of it, you'll be A-OK. The cookies and milk to your left are proof of that. When I was first diagnosed with over 200 allergies and intolerances, I knew safe cookies would be a challenge. So go forth and conquer the big three.

I hope these recipes are a blessing to you and your loved ones. If you ever need help, feel free to reach out. If we're not able to help you, I'm sure we can point you in the right direction. I wish you all happy and safe eating!

Your Friend In The Kitchen,
Kathlena
~The Allergy Chef :)

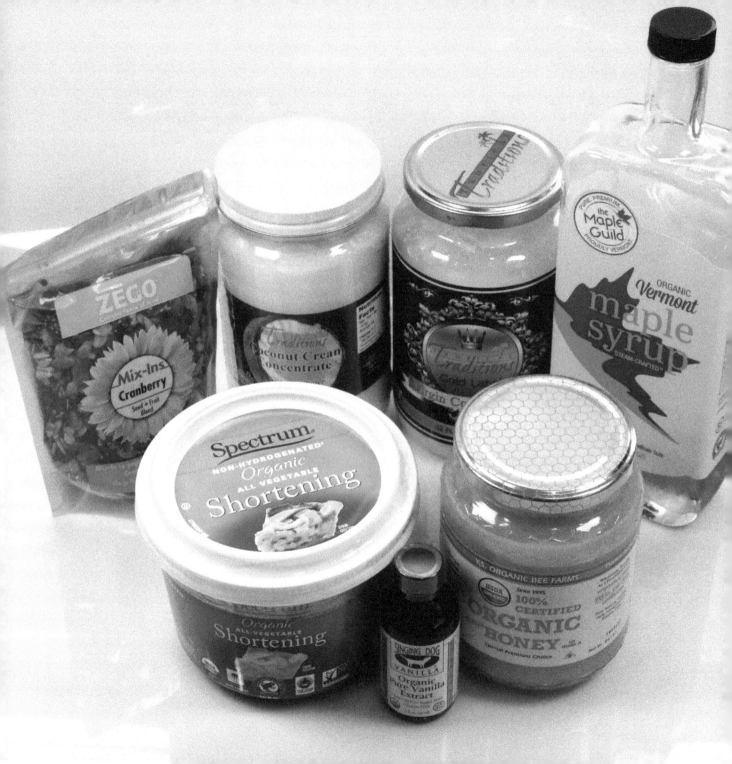

Building A Safe Pantry

When first being diagnosed with any form of food allergy or intolerance, it can be incredibly difficult to find safe food and build a pantry that you're comfortable with. Your food journal will help you keep track of what's safe for you, so make sure you stay on top of it. Don't be afraid to call companies and ask a million questions. If you feel they lack transparency, perhaps it's not worth eating the food. Photographed are some corn free items that we keep in stock (I don't currently use all of them due to the number of allergies and intolerances I have). On page 17, there are two links that you corn free folks will find very helpful. On the following pages, there are lots of brands listed in parenthesis that are great for those of you with a corn allergy. Additionally, we've included a list of companies that are allergy friendly, and a list of companies that are top 8 allergy free as well. All of these lists were accurate as of July, 2018. Anytime you see a list or series of suggestions, still do your due diligence. For example, one of the suggestions we make is Once Again Sunflower Seed Butter. This is safe for a corn allergic IF you're able to tolerate food made in a shared facility with nuts. If not, you'll need to make your own seed butters at home. Why? Because the leading brand of Sunflower Seed Butter (that's top 8 free, yay!) uses corn derivatives in some of their products. I say that to share with you that it's all one HUGE flow chart. Some of you can have A, while others need B. No one can have C, and everyone longs for D. Finally, when trying new things, don't be afraid to call a company and ask for a sample. Let them know about your allergies, and that you would like to try before buying. If it works out for you, be sure to purchase extra :)

Pictured: Spectrum Organic Shortening, Singing Dog Organic Vanilla Extract, YS Raw Organic Honey, Zego Mix-Ins, Tropical Traditions Coconut Cream, Tropical Traditions Coconut Oil, The Maple Guild Organic Maple Syrup (steam-crafted, no defoamer)

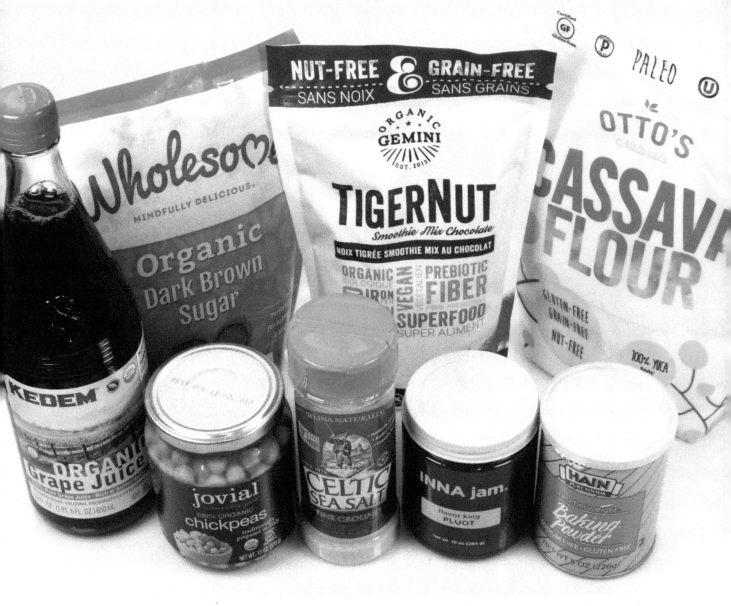

Pictured: Jovial Organic Chickpeas, Celtic Sea Salt, Inna Jam Plout Jam, Hain Featherweight Baking Powder, Kedem Organic Grape Juice, Wholesome Sweeteners Organic Dark Brown Sugar, Organic Gemini Tiger Nut Flour (not a nut, tuber vegetable), Otto's Cassava Flour

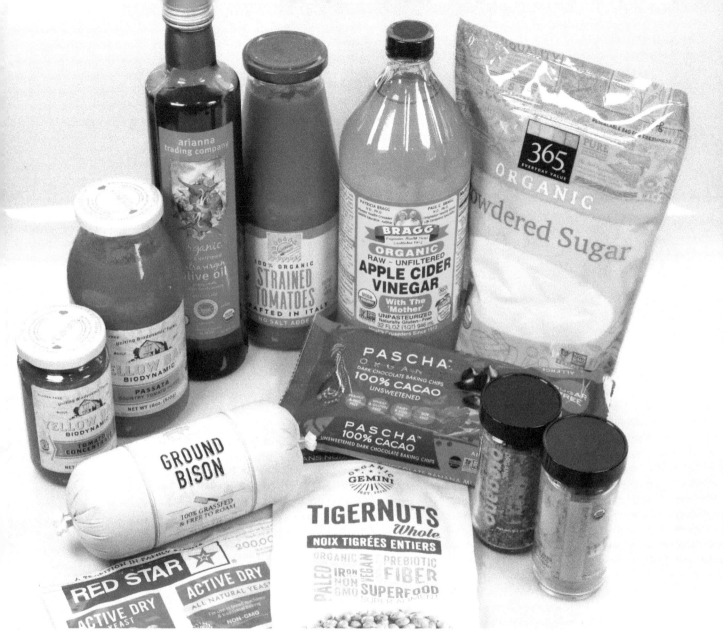

...tured: Red Star Yeast, Organic Gemini Whole Tiger Nuts, The Honest Bison Ground Bison, Spicely Organics ...yme, Spicely Organics Onion Granules, Pascha Organic Dark Chocolate Chips (100% cacao), Yellow Barn ...ganic Tomato Concentrate, Yellow Barn Organic Tomato Sauce, Safe Olive Oil (recently unavailable), Bio Nature ...ained Tomatoes, Bragg Organic Apple Cider Vinegar, 365 (Whole Foods Brand) Organic Powdered Sugar.

Common Top 8 & Corn Free Ingredients

Here are a list of items you will come across in the book, or things we love to keep on hand in our kitchen. In parenthesis are brands that were corn free as of 7/2018.

Flours & Baking
Sorghum Flour (Authentic Foods)
Potato Starch (Authentic Foods)
Tapioca Starch (Authentic Foods)
Arrowroot Starch/Flour (Authentic Foods)
Baking Powder (Hain Featherweight)
Baking Soda (Arm & Hammer)
Cassava Flour (Otto's Naturals)
Gluten Free Rolled Oats (glutenfreeoats.com)
Gluten Free Oat Flour (glutenfreeoats.com)
Organic Gemini Tiger Nut Flour (tuber, not nut)

Chocolates
Raw Organic Cacao Powder (Hummingbird)
Pascha Organic Dark Chocolate

Sweeteners
Raw Organic Sugar
Organic Sugar (Kirkland/Costco)
Organic Powdered Sugar (365/Whole Foods)
Organic Light & Dark Brown Sugars
Organic Maple Sugar (Hummingbird)
Raw Organic Honey (YS, Local)

Seasonings
Sea Salt (Celtic)
Pink Himalayan Salt
Organic Onion Granules (Spicely Organic)
Organic Garlic Granules (Spicely Organic)
Organic Dill Weed (Spicely Organic)
Organic Parsley (Spicely Organic)
Organic Ground Ginger (Spicely Organic)
Organic Ground Mustard (Spicely Organic)

Organic Black Pepper (Spicely Organic)
Organic Ground Cinnamon (Spicely Organic)
Organic Ground Nutmeg (Spicely Organic)
Organic Ground Cloves (Spicely Organic)
Organic Raw Ground Vanilla Bean (Singing Dog)
Organic Smoked Paprika (Spicely Organic)
Organic Apple Cider Vinegar (Bragg)
Yeast (Red Star)

Extracts & Flavors
Organic Vanilla Extract (Singing Dog)
Organic Orange Oil (Veriditas Botanicals)
Organic Peppermint Oil (Veriditas Botanicals)
Organic Lemon Oil (Veriditas Botanicals)

Milk & Butter
Organic Unsweetened Milk (Homemade)
Organic Shortening (Spectrum)

Nuts & Seeds
Organic Chia Seeds (Black & White)
Golden Flax Seeds (Namaste)
Organic Pumpkin Seeds
Mix-Ins (Zego)

Dried Fruit
Organic Raw Medjool Dates
Organic Raisins

Pasta
Organic Rice Pasta (Lundberg)
Organic Black Bean Pasta (Tolerant)
Organic Lentil Pasta (Tolerant)

Fruits & Vegetables
Local is best, as you'll be able to ask lots of questions about how it's grown, processed, stored, etc. While frozen and canned can be found, the success rates will vary. Concerns when selecting fresh produce would be waxes, which can be corn based, as well as cleaners and storage. Localharvest.org is a great starting place, as many locations offer shipping (corn free bananas anyone?). With fruit, there are some that will be next to impossible to find corn free in grocery stores, including pineapple and bananas. These will take a LOT of research, and you will most likely need to convince a farmer to ship them to you. I've personally had pineapple once in the past 5 years, and I'm grateful everyday he was willing to ship to me that one time.

Meat*
Before selecting meat, you'll need to determine how severe your corn allergy is. For some of us, we can't consume the meat of animals that have been fed corn. Personally, I'm one of those people. It greatly limits my options, however, I've found that farmers in the Pacific Northwest offer better options year-round.

Once you've figured out the feed issue, you'll have to determine the processing issue. The FDA has regulations on how meat must be processed, and some of the options are bad for corn allergics. Finally, you'll need to figure out the packaging. Soaker pads don't have a good track record for people with severe corn allergies. In my case, I've been able to find options where the meat is packaged in non-corn based package without any soaking materials. More often than not, you won't be able to find that in most grocery stores, even when purchasing a case from the manufacturer.

One last meat tip: don't purchase ground meat from a grocery store. There's a higher chance of contamination from other products. If you must, get a meat grinder (or stand mixer attachment) to grind meat at home.

Bison (The Honest Bison)
North Star Bison

Further Resources
Take the time to get VERY familiar with corn derivatives, which are used in the manufacturing of foods, and also as ingredients.
https://web.archive.org/web/20160304001706/http://www.cornallergens.com/list/corn-allergen-list.php

Here is an old (2014) list of foods that were at one point considered to be truly corn free. You'll need to keep a food journal to ensure foods are safe for you. This list is an awesome starting point, but be sure to do your due diligence.
http://corn-freefoods.blogspot.com/2014/07/corn-free-foods-products-list-july-2014.html

Let's Talk About Brand Names

You'll notice in the book I'll often say "of your choice" meaning you should use a brand that's safe for you. Since starting our bakery, we have learned A LOT about shared facilities and cross contamination. Here's some tips I can pass on to you:

- Bob's Red Mill isn't safe for people with a nut, soy, or corn allergy. The hit and miss ratio simply isn't worth it in my opinion.
- Authentic Foods is super awesome. They sell flour, and are safe even for corn allergics.
- GlutenFreeOats.com are the only top 8 free, organic, beyond gluten free, and corn free oats that I know of.
- Check your local Costco and make phone calls with the item number. They have several items that come from a top 8 free facility.
- The 365 Whole Foods brand of Organic Maple Syrup comes from a top 8 free facility.
- We buy the wholesale bag of Otto's Cassava Flour, and it's processed in the white zone of their facility. It's safe for top 8, and corn free too.
- We use Organic Gemini Tiger Nut Flour without any issues.
- Singing Dog vanilla extract is top 8 free, and the alcohol is derived from cane sugar.
- Wholesome Sweeteners is a great source of top 8 free facility sugars.

There are other brands that we are aware of which are mentioned throughout the book, but more than anything, you have to read all of the labels. As of the printing of this book, companies are not legally required to disclose if their product was made in shared facility with or on shared equipment with allergens. This is why we make it a point to call regularly, even with trusted brands. For example, Frontier CoOp, maker of Simply Organic, is a facility that's shared with every major allergen. And don't stop at asking about the final product. Ask about each ingredient in the product, and the packaging as well. We called Follow Your Heart once to ask about their egg free replacer. Turns out, the source ingredients were made on shared equipment with several major allergens, and they didn't declare it. They went on to tell me that they did in-house testing of their products... As someone who strives to keep others safe, I found this to be unacceptable, and we discontinued the use of their product.

Once you find a good product, buy several, especially of the same lot. It's one of the easiest ways to make sure you always have safe food in the house.

Notes When Ordering & Purchasing Food

When purchasing food for people with food allergies, the first tip I can give you is: don't touch the bulk bins. People have their hands in and out of them, and you have no idea where they've been. However, bulk and case ordering is totally in your best interest. You also need to know a little more about the food industry... There's an awesome company that we order from called Hummingbird Naturals. They sell items that come from top 8 free producers. However, you'd have to be in the know to know that they receive 50 pound bags and repackage them into 5 pound bags... alongside major allergens. The only way to have the top 8 free products is to order 50 pound bags. The same goes for other companies. For example, Otto's (cassava) has a white zone where they package certain sizes, and those are the ones that will be safe for a corn allergic. Feel free to call them directly to order such items.

For those of you that are here for the corn free elements, avoid biodegradable like the plague. Not all BD items are made from corn, but so many are. Also, some plastics are corn derived. You will have to do a lot of investigating. There are companies like Zego that go the extra mile for the corn free community, and they've ensured their packaging is safe too.

Don't be scared off by a company who may sell a product you're allergic to. Many of them have multiple facilities. However, the only way to know is to call. Finally, you'll notice that just about everything we use is organic. That's done by design for our household (many reasons). While I'm sure there are many conventional brands that are safe, we feel that people with food allergies, intolerances, and special diets are usually needing food that's clean, high quality, and nutrient dense.

Our Favorite Top 8 Allergy Free Products

The US Top 8 Allergens are: Wheat, Dairy, Egg, Soy, Peanut, Tree Nuts, Fish, and Shell Fish.

The products /brands listed below are free from the top 8 allergens, and most of the facilities are dedicated (at the time of this writing). It's important to note that larger companies have multiple facilities. They may have some products that meet your needs, and others that don't. It's why it's critical that you do research and make phone calls before introducing new items if you're living with severe food allergies. In the case of our allergy kid, he has reactions off-and-on to foods made in shared facilities and on shared equipment with his allergens. We have adopted a strict policy of nothing shared when purchasing food for him. In the long run, it means we make a lot of food from scratch, but his safety is worth it. On the other hand, he's intolerant to eggs (not allergic) so we allow foods that may be made in a shared space with eggs, such as Little Northern Bakehouse. You will have to keep a food journal and monitor reactions closely when making these sorts of decisions for yourself and your children.

365 (Whole Foods) - Some Products

88 Acres (Snacks, Seed Butters)

Arm & Hammer

Authentic Foods (Flours)

Better Bites (Dessert)

Cooks Organics (Extracts)

Crofters Organic (Jams & Jellies)

Cybele's Free To Eat (Cookies, Pasta)

Earth Balance

Enjoy Life Foods (Chocolate, Snacks, Cookies)

Free 2 Be (Granola Bars, Candies)

GF Harvest (GlutenFreeOats.com)

Glee Gum (Corn and Soy Lecithin in Facility, Not On Lines)

GoldThread

Hidden Star Orchard

Hilary's Eat Well (Some Products)

Inna (Jams & Preserves)

Jacob's Farm (Produce)

Jo Organic Coffee

Jovial Organic Chickpeas (Excellent for Aquafaba)

Karen's Naturals (Freeze Dried)

Kirkland Organics (Costco) - Some Items

Libre Naturals (granola, snacks)

Lundberg Farms (Rice Only Products)

Namaste Foods (Raw Materials, Box Mixes)

No Whey Chocolates (Candies)

Organic Gemini (Tiger Nuts, not a nut, some products contain coconut)

Otto's Naturals (Cassava)

Piping Gourmet (Frozen Treats)

Pomona (Pectin)

Real Pickles

Shady Maple Farms

Singing Dog Vanilla

Spicely Organics (Seasonings)

Sun Butter

Surf Sweets (Candies)

The Date Lady (Coconut Products Use Separate Equipment)

The Ginger People (Some Products)

The Honest Bison

The Maple Guild

Townsend Farms (Frozen Fruit)

Veriditas Botanicals (Oils)

Vermont Village (Apple & Vinegar Products)

Wild Zora Foods (Each Flavor Has Separate Equipment, One Flavor Contains Allergens)

YS Honey

Zego Snacks (Bars and Granola)

More Allergy Friendly Brands

Some items are top 8 free, but the facility or line may not be. Some items contain one or more of the top 8 allergens, but may be a good fit for your family.

Seasonings & Flavorings

India Tree

Ojio

Milk & Butter

Daiya

Follow Your Heart

Kite Kill

Myioko's

Tofutti

Snacks

18 Rabbits

Cascadian Farms

Clif Kids

Epic Bar

Go Raw

Home Free Treats

Junkless Snacks

Kettle (Chips)

Kind Bar

Kinnikinnick

Nature's Path

North Coast

Rule Breaker Snacks

Siete Foods

Simple Mills

Udi's

Pantry

Eden Organics

Edward & Sons

Jovial Foods

Lotus Foods

Once Again

Organicville

San-J

Sir Kensington's

Tinkyada

Frozen

365 (Vegetables)

Ian's Natural Foods

So Delicious

Wholly Wholesome

All About Substitutions - Eggs

Eggs are a common ingredient in baking, and it's important to know why. Eggs are a binder, can be used as a leavening agent, and can also add moisture to your recipe. They're also very nutritious. If you can't have eggs, here are several options that all "equal" one egg that you can find online and in books when doing your research. I'll come back to those quotation marks in a moment.

1 TBSP Ground Flax + 3 TBSP Water
1 TBSP Chia Seeds + 1/3 cup Water
1 TBSP Soy Protein + 3 TBSP Water
1 TBSP Agar Agar + 1 TBSP Water
2 TBSP Arrowroot Flour
2 TBSP Potato Starch
1/2 Ripe, Smashed Banana
1/4 cup Unsweetened Applesauce
3 TBSP Peanut Butter
Commercial egg replacer such as Ener-G, Namaste, Follow Your Heart, or Daiya brands

Each of these should "equal" one egg, but in all honesty, they never really do. As you get into egg free baking, especially if you are also DF and GF, things just don't work the way conventional recipes do. Our kids have gotten use to cookies that crumble, and simply accept this as a fact of life. In the past, we had awesome results with: **Potato Starch, Chia Seeds, and DF Milk mixed together as a replacement. Now, we use Namaste Golden Flax**. Some recipes in this book will use our original combination. The draw back is that chia can sometimes lend a texture and taste you don't want. To combat this, I also use potato starch and milk mixed together as a replacement. The key on the flax is to use the right brand. Not all brands gel the same way, which was a problem we ran into.

All About Substitutions - Dairy

Dairy is a common ingredient in baking and cooking. Cow's milk is creamy, and doesn't have much flavor. This makes it very useful for sweet and savory cooking and baking. What makes it better than water is the texture, and general makeup.

Dairy substitutions are simple. You can use rice, soy, almond, hemp, hazelnut, oat, and coconut milk alternatives. Rice milk is thin, beware. Soy is close to the thickness of milk, but we don't like it given the soy issues in this country. Almond milk works well, and we prefer to use organic unsweetened almond milk. Hemp is simply odd in taste. Hazelnut milk has a strong flavor, so it may not work well in all recipes. Coconut milk is nice and thick. It can work well, but does have a distinct flavor unlike some of the other choices. Currently, we use an organic oat milk that we make fresh at home. More than anything, experiment and see which one you like best!

All About Substitutions - Wheat

A note about how we use flour. As previously mentioned, Kid Two requires a special food rotation, so when putting together new recipes for him, I purposefully use single flours rather than a blend. Most GF flours contain rice, which we avoid so he can have rice with other meals. If you don't need a rotation, you should try using your safe/go-to flour of choice in place of ours, and you may even have better results. Part of the reason store-bought blends work is because of the texture combinations, as well as the xantham gum etc. that's added. For us, with my severe corn allergy, xantham gum usually isn't allowed in the house.

To All of My Friends With a Corn Allergy

If corn is your only allergy, then you'll need to source safe eggs and dairy. If you have a severe corn allergy, you may find that eating the products of animals fed corn can cause problems for you, even though "it's not supposed to". You may reach a point where you need to do lots of research to find safe farms in your area. You may also be able to find a farmer willing to mail you frozen goods. If you live in the PA area, the Amish are an amazing resource. There are also great farms in Oregon.

If you have a dairy and corn allergy, and can tolerate nuts or oats, you may be better off making your own milk. Be sure to use a corn free nut milk bag. If you can't have eggs and corn, the potato starch and chia seed egg substitute still works, however, you'll need to find safe potato starch and chia.

All About Substitutions - Reversing It
(For People Without Food Allergies)

So you don't have food allergies, but you have the book? Awesomesauce! Here are some tips for you.

Wheat & Grains

Gluten free baking requires a combination of more than one pseudo-grain to create what should be wheat flour. In your case, you're looking for sorghum, potato, and arrowroot listed in a recipe. Those are the replacements. You'll add up the total amount used, then sub in wheat flour instead. If you use something that contains more than wheat, such as xantham gum, then you would take out any gums we call for, such as guar.

Milk & Butter

These are the easiest in my opinion. It's a one-for-one substitution rate. See. Painless.

Eggs

Throughout the recipes, you'll see a note that says egg substitute, or you may see an instruction to combine potato starch and almond milk. These are the eggs. 2 TBSP of potato starch is roughly one egg. If I call for 4 TBSP of potato + milk, you would use 2 eggs instead.

Example

1 1/2 cup White Sorghum Flour
1/2 cup Organic Buckwheat Flour
1/3 cup Potato Starch
1/3 cup Arrowroot Starch
4 tsp Baking Powder

You would use 2 2/3 cups of flour of your choosing. I suggest start at the 2 cup mark, then add in 1/3 at a time to make sure it's necessary.

A Few More Thoughts...

If you're not keeping a detailed food journal, start today. Over time, it will help you understand the patterns that are unique to you. The journal also becomes an amazing aid at diagnosing any other medical conditions you may be suffering with. It will help your GP/Allergist/Specialist hone in on what could be the cause, and also help when selecting test to run.

If you're here for the top 8 allergy free element of the book, everything here works perfectly for you. In some cases, there will be less expensive brands that you can purchase since corn is not part of your equation.

I'm often asked if "it's safe to see what my corn allergic child can handle"... I'm not a doctor, and I can't give medical advice. What I can share with parents however is how painful allergic reactions can be. Just because it's not anaphylaxis doesn't mean it's all roses and rainbows. I will often share with parents that if their child is under the age of 10, please refrain from experimenting on them. They won't be able to communicate effectively with you to let you know 6 hours after ingestion that something is wrong. If the child is over the age of 10, and is an excellent communicator, let them choose. For some kids, they're content with the safety of their food. For others, they want to know what their limits are. I'm personally not a fan of subjecting others to unnecessary pain and discomfort, especially when I know first hand what they're going through.

Is this life hard? Oh my goodness yes. Will there be days where all you want to do is scream and cry and get angry at the food industry? Why, yes of course. Your feelings are totally valid. However, once the feeling has passed, you have to get back to business because someone is counting on you to stay strong and make sure there's something safe to eat. You CAN do this. Our family is living proof that not only can you do this, you can have fun with it, and thrive.

Tips For The Recipes

Tips about dairy free butter.
In the past, we had great experiences with Earth Balance Vegan Buttery Sticks, which contains soy. We prefer this brand because it's not made in a shared facility with dairy, which Kid Two is severely allergic to. This brand also makes Soy Free Butter, and what we currently use - the Food Service Box. It is a 30 pound box and needs to be special ordered. It's top 8 free, but does contain corn derivatives. You can also consider using Spectrum Shortening or experiment with olive oil, coconut oil, or tiger nut oil (tiger nut is a tuber vegetable).

We don't use beef.
Kid Two and I are both allergic to beef. Anytime bison is used in the book, both beef and turkey would be a great 1:1 selection as well.

If you are allergic to nuts and dairy, you may need to make your own milk at home.
We make fresh organic oat milk at home because of the bakery we started. It was the only way to guarantee a dairy free milk that wasn't made in a shared facility with any of the top 8. Pacific Foods has great Organic dairy free milks, but they're made in a shared facility. They have good practices and standards, but I wouldn't chance it if you are severely allergic. They also make an oat milk, but cannot guarantee it's gluten free due to the growing conditions.

It's Simple so you CAN Substitute.
You may notice some of the recipes are simple, or don't use store-bought flour blends. This allows for easier personalized substitution based on your needs. We know that no two people with allergies are the same, so we encourage you to change things when necessary.

Prep, Freeze, and Freeze!
Many of the recipes can be frozen and used again later. Sometimes it's the batter that you freeze, other times, the whole dish. If you have more than one child, or live a busy life, freezing items should become an awesome part of your kitchen routine.

You NEED a Kitchen Scale
Many of our recipes use weighted measurements for accuracy, and improved outcome for readers. You'll need a kitchen scale. You can get a nice digital one on Amazon for $10.

Lingo & Basic Tools

There are several tools that we use almost daily, and some common lingo you should be aware of.

tsp & t are both short for teaspoon

TBSP & T are both short for Tablespoon. There are 3t in 1T.

c is short for cup.

GF = Gluten Free, DF = Dairy free, EF = Egg Free, NF = Nut Free, CF = Corn Free

Room Temp, usually referring to butter and eggs, means allow the ingredient to sit out so it's no longer chilled. With butter, it should be easy to press with a finger (soft), but not melted.

Small and Medium Cookie Dough Scooper. We use the OXO brand, and they are simply awesome. The small scooper holds 2t and the medium holds 1.5T. There's also a large one, but we use an ice cream scooper for bigger scoops.

Good measuring cups and spoons for both wet and dry ingredients. We like the OXO brand for dry goods because it's accurate. I once bought a set online, and they didn't measure up. Literally :)

A good blender. We have a Vitamix. It's great for blending, easy to clean, and simply wonderful.

A good stand mixer. We have a Kitchen Aid. We simply couldn't live without ours. You can mix by hand, but a good stand mixer will make things go much faster.

Scissors. I use regularly to open packages, etc. We keep 2 sets for food items, 3 for baking, and 1 utility pair in the kitchen. Why so many? With all the allergies, we wash them after each use to prevent cross contamination.

Time To Invest

So you have a lot of food allergies, or are a severe corn allergic? No problem. We live in a modern time where there are so many awesome tools available that you can be up and running in no time.

For those who are new to this world that come to us with a long list of allergens, I often tell them a little story: A couple of years ago we finally finished our taxes and learned that we had spent $32,000 on food. That's a CAR. A nice one! That was for 6 people, 5 of which had food allergies and/or a special diet.

That happened around the time we officially launched our business, and thankfully, most of our food is now a write off since we use it to develop recipes for others. However, we've had to sacrifice a lot to feed our family. I went 6 years without purchasing a new pair of shoes, and Karlton will only buy a new pair if holes develop in his. We don't eat out very often, vacations are staycations, and frugal is simply how we live. However, on the flip side, we have every tool and appliance necessary to make our kitchen run smoothly. No two families, or budgets, are the same. You'll need to find a balance that works for you. In our case, our medical bills went to just about nothing as soon as we had everyone's food issues properly diagnosed, and there's where a good amount of the funds came from. However, Karlton works 3 jobs to pull in enough income for our family. Ouch. His dedication to providing for us is nothing short of amazing.

So what do you need to invest in? Everything. When you're newly diagnosed, it's suggested that you replace pots, pans, utensils, and anything porous. If you live in a mixed allergen household, you may need two sets (we have three sets) of a lot of items. We also have things like a great blender, stand mixer, NutraMilk machine, ice cream machine (with a compressor built in, no bowl freezing), sno-cone machine, food processor, multi-functioning pressure cooker, rice cooker, tortilla press (cooks and presses at the same time), three toaster ovens, SodaStream (glass), air fryer, and juicer. At some point, we'll also be adding a small scale deep fryer, pasta making items, and doubling up on select appliances for my personal use. You can see how that can all add up quickly, however, we've made it a top priority in our home.

I say all of that to encourage you. If there's something you want to make safely at home, most likely, there's a tool that can help you succeed. In some cases, you don't need a fancy machine (looking at you bread maker) and in other cases, you'll be so happy each time you pull out your ice cream maker and have something tasty in an hour. Plan and budget for these expenses, especially if you are feeding young children with allergies, so they can enjoy all sorts of foods.

Kindness & Compassion

OK, I'm going to try to make this my final "one more thought" :)

Kindness and compassion are so critical when interacting with people living with food allergies. Reactions can manifest in numerous ways, and no two people are the same. For corn allergics, there are some of us that suffer from Corn Rage. It's not common, but for those of us that get it, we understand... You can go from being as happy as a clam to ready to put your fist through a wall in a matter of minutes. When I say rage, I mean RAGE. It's not done on purpose, and it's incredibly difficult to control. I say that as an adult... could you image how tough it must be for a kid or teen? I am so blessed to have a family that shows me kindness and compassion on bad days. However, I make sure that bad days are few and far between. I don't take risks, eat strange food, etc. I am diligent in making sure food is as safe as possible to prevent problems from happening.

We have also seen this issue in our Low/No Sugar kid. Recently, he had an evening where he was fine, and then just wasn't. I mean it was BAD. That's when I realized we had tried a new item at dinner time for him that was low/no sugar, but not good for him. In that moment, I calmly said to him, "I'm pretty sure the food you ate is getting to you. I'm going to give you one chance to shut your mouth and walk away. Go to your bed and read or go to sleep. If you don't want this opportunity, you will be in a lot of trouble because you are out of control." I was calm and slow. He heard me, and agreed, and walked away. The next day, it had cleared his system and he was totally fine. We talked about food, and how it effects him, and I apologized for the dinner I had made, and promised we wouldn't be using that brand ever again.

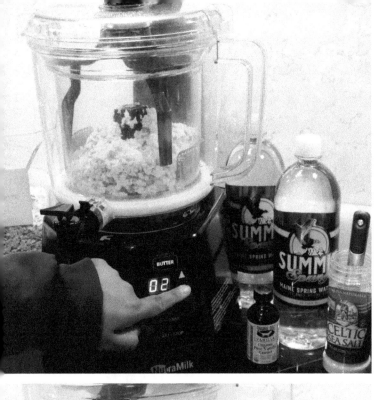
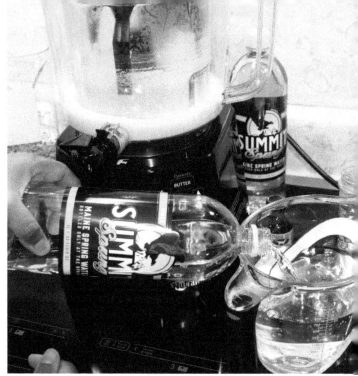
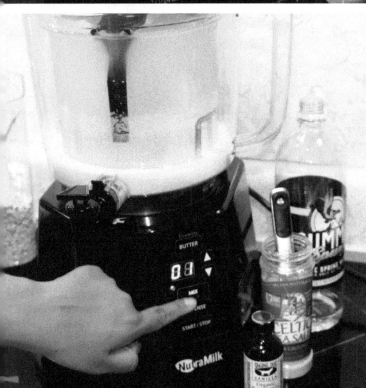
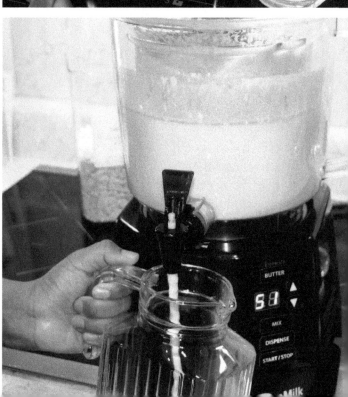

The Important of The Basics

When you reach a point where you need to make most of your food from scratch, you'll need to master the basics. With them, you'll be able to make just about anything you could ever want. When living with a corn allergy, or needing to be free from the top 8 allergens, there's a good chance you won't be able to find a safe commercial milk/non-dairy milk option that's safe. You may struggle to find other basics such as sauces, condiments, and everything in between. Soon you will find yourself grinding your own meat at home, sourcing bones for homemade broth, making granolas, cookies, bread, and well, everything you won't be able to purchase in stores. I don't say that to deter you, rather, to encourage you. With the right tools (see page 28), you'll be up an running in no time. To the left is the wonderful NutraMilk. While you can make non-dairy milks with a blender and nut-milk bag, we've found that the NutraMilk offers speed and a LOT of efficiency. Our yield has more than doubled with this machine. We use it for our bakery, and for my corn free tiger nut milk. Before the machine, I wasn't able to have any milk, as tiger nuts are so incredibly hard, and the blender wasn't able to handle them. Now, there's always milk on tap. Why is that so important? Because with milk you can create ice cream, yogurt, pancakes, waffles, cream sauce, richer smoothies, baked goods, and more. So let's dive in to a few of my favorite basics. Save $50 when you purchase one with the code TheAllergyChef.

Oat Milk & Tiger Nut Milk

Vegan, Top 8 Free, Free From: Gluten, Cane Sugar, Coconut, Corn, Legumes, Mustard, Nightshades, Seeds, Sesame, Sulfites

Friendly To: AIP, Paleo, Low Histamine

For AIP & Paleo, use Tiger Nut Milk

I can't tell you enough just how much I love that we can make our own milk. It truly is a game changer. The directions below are for use in a NutraMilk. You can use a blender + nut milk bath method for oat milk. Given the hardness of tiger nuts, you will need a NutraMilk or AlmondCow.

Oat Milk Ingredients:

140g Gluten Free Oats

4 cups Safe Water

1 tsp Organic Vanilla Extract

1/2 tsp Celtic Sea Salt

Tiger Nut Milk Ingredients:

150g Whole Tiger Nuts, soaked overnight

4 cups Safe Water

Oat Milk Directions:

Soak your oats for 20 minutes, then drain off any excess liquid. Add the oats to your NutraMilk and start the butter mode for 2 minutes. Next, add your other ingredients, then start the blend mode on the default 1 minute setting. Finally, start the dispense mode and capture all of your delicious milk.

Tiger Nut Milk Directions:

Soak your tiger nuts in safe water overnight, then drain off the excess liquid. Place the tiger nuts in your NutraMilk and start the butter mode for 2 minutes. Next, add you water, and start the blend mode for the default 1 minute. Finally, start the dispense mode. I personally like to place a nut milk bag over the mouth of my container when capturing tiger nut milk to remove excess pulp.

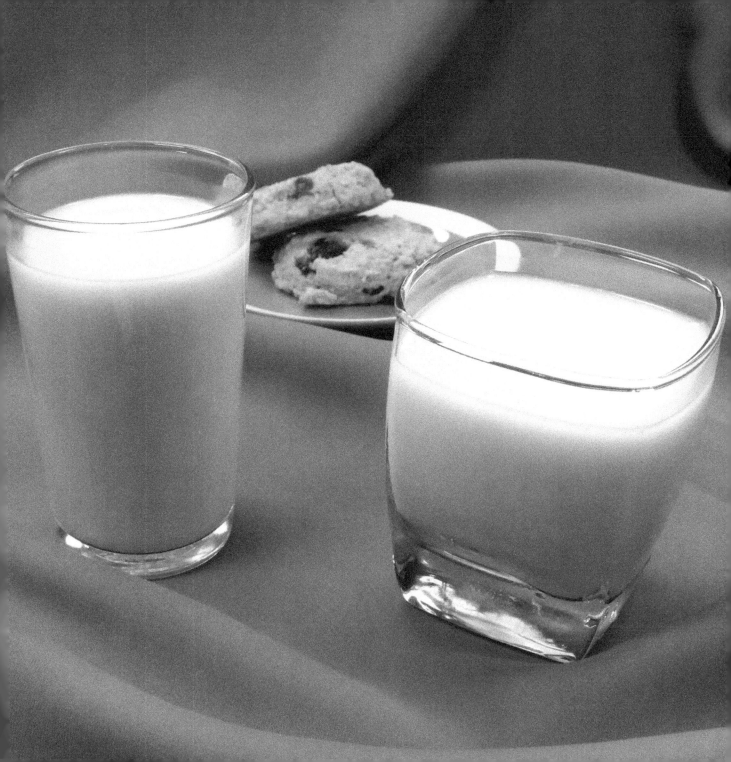

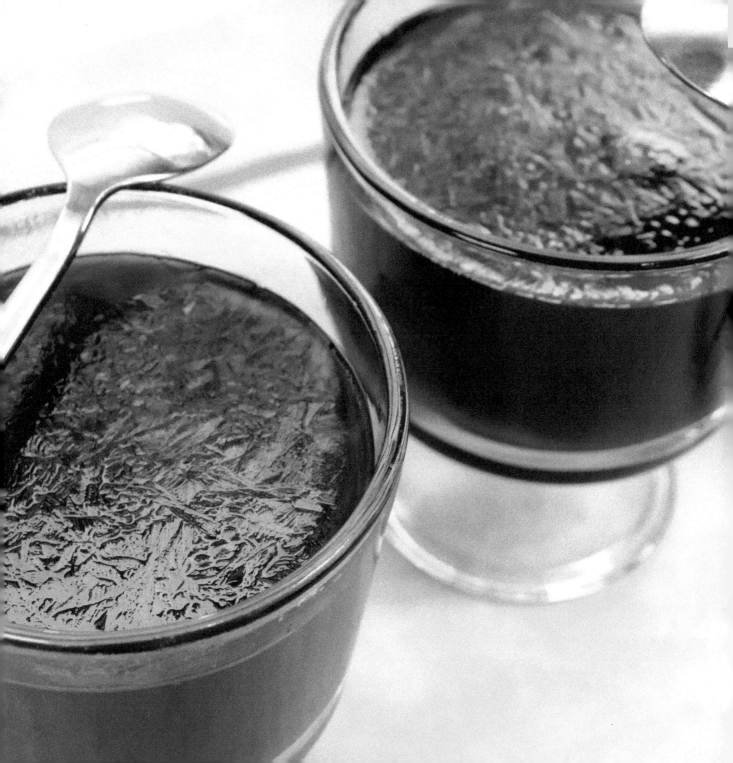

Grape Juice Slushie

Vegan, Top 8 Free, Free From: Gluten, Cane Sugar, Coconut, Corn, Legumes, Mustard, Nightshades, Seeds, Sesame, Sulfites

Friendly To: AIP, Paleo, Low Histamine

This is the only way I take my grape juice: as a slushie. For those of you who may be AIP, or who struggle with sugar, make small slushies. Grape juice, in my opinion, is naturally high in sugar.

Ingredients:

Kedem Grape Juice

Directions:

This is so simple, yet SO rewarding. Pour grape juice into a glass cup and freeze. The size of the cup will determine how long you will need to freeze for. You don't want your juice to freeze solid, rather, lightly frozen, easy to pierce with a fork or spoon. The result is magic.

Maple Slushie

Vegan, Top 8 Free, Free From: Gluten, Cane Sugar, Coconut, Corn, Legumes, Mustard, Nightshades, Seeds, Sesame, Sulfites

Friendly To: AIP, Paleo, Low Histamine

The kids have told me that this dish tastes phenomenal. It works well as a pot pie filling, or as a pasta/rice topping. You can also serve this over cauliflower rice or zoodles.

Ingredients:

Safe Water

Organic Maple Syrup

About Maple Syrup
When it comes to reading a food label, never judge a book by its cover, or take it at face value. Companies omit processing aids, defoamers, cleaners, etc. The Maple Guild is the only company I've ever found that doesn't use a defoamer product. Rather, they use their own cold maple sap as the defoamer, rather than sunflower, safflower, cream, etc.

Directions:

Another super simple, yet VERY rewarding treat to make. Here's how I usually make my slushies:

Remove several ounces from your bottle of safe water. Add a your desired amount of maple syrup (we all experience sweet differently). Freeze. When the slushie is just right, it will look almost cloudy. There won't be solid chunks of ice that have formed yet.

Alternatively, you can put your maple water in a glass cup as pictured and freeze.

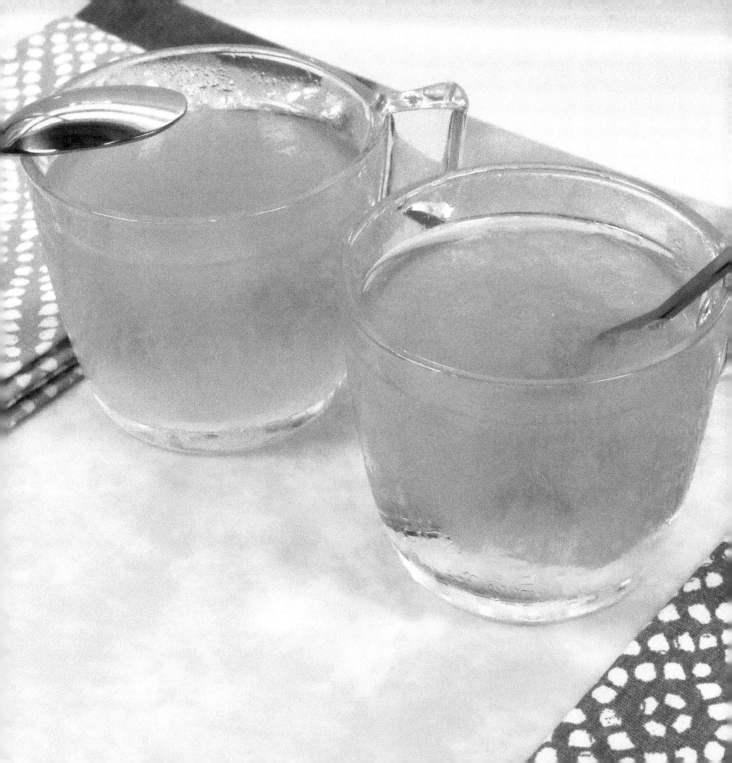

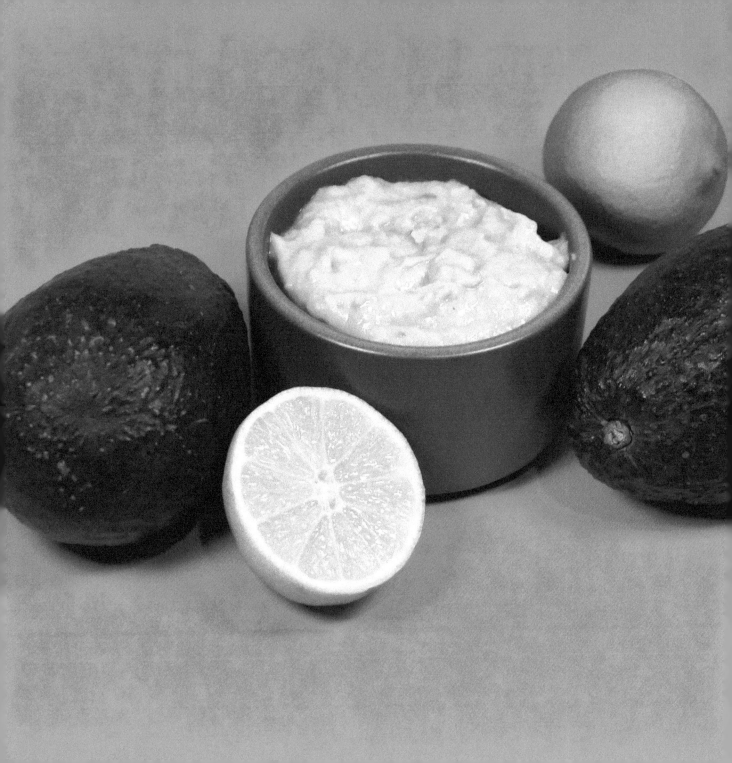

Creamy Avocado Sauce

Vegan, Top 8 Free, Free From: Gluten, Cane Sugar, Coconut, Corn, Legumes, Mustard, Nightshades, Seeds, Sesame, Sulfites

Friendly To: AIP, Paleo

Compatible With: Low Histamine

Safe Sourcing Notes: We are blessed to live near Brokaw (Will's) Avocados. I call Will about once every 6 weeks to order a case of spray free avocado. When they come in from the trees, he puts them straight into a box for me, free from any ripening gas, which is corn derived. As of 7/2018 he is no longer shipping, but open to doing so in the future, so send him an email and ask for future updates. Until then, research and find yourself a grower that's willing to help you. For the limes, we have a few local farms that don't place wax on their citrus fruits.

One could argue this is a hop skip and jump away from guacamole, and I certainly wouldn't argue. It's delicious with tortillas, chips, and tacos. Everyone in the house absolutely loves this sauce.

Ingredients:

9 ounces Avocado Flesh

3.5 ounces Organic Purple Onion

3 ounces Tiger Nut Milk

3/4 tsp Celtic Sea Salt

1/2 Lime, squeezed (omit for Low Histamine)

Directions:

Cut open your avocado, remove the seeds, and add to your food processor. The hass variety is suggested. Add all of the other ingredients, and finally, squeeze half of your lime into the processor. Pulse your processor until a smooth sauce forms.

Ketchup

Vegan, Top 8 Free, Free From: Gluten, Cane Sugar, Coconut, Corn, Legumes, Mustard, Seeds, Sesame, Sulfites

Friendly To: Paleo

If you're like us and have to make so many things from scratch, have fun with it. Take the time to create your own labels for the full ketchup experience :)

Ingredients:

7.5 ounces Tomato Concentrate (Yellow Barn)

3 TBSP Safe Water

2 tsp Organic Maple Syrup (Maple Guild)

2 tsp Organic Apple Cider Vinegar (Bragg)

1 tsp Organic Onion Granules (Spicely Organic)

1/2 tsp Celtic Sea Salt

Directions:

Combine all of your ingredients together in a bowl or small sauce pan. You can use a whisk or fork. Mix until smooth. You can store this in the fridge in a squeeze bottle for easy use, or in a glass jar.

This ketchup tastes delicious not only on fries, but on meatballs too :)

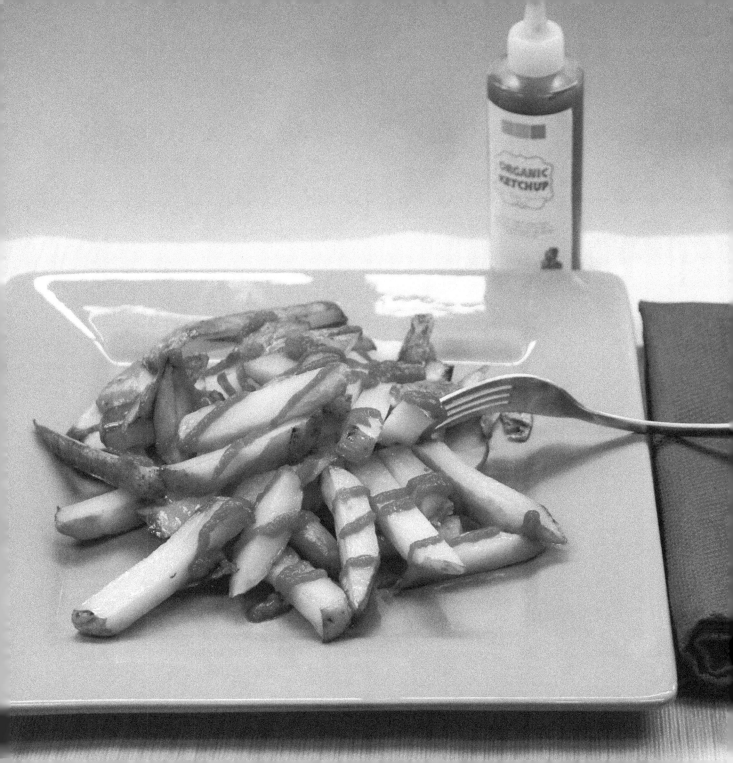

Pesto

Vegan, Top 8 Free, Free From: Gluten, Cane Sugar, Coconut, Corn, Legumes, Mustard, Nightshades, Seeds, Sesame, Sulfites
Friendly To: AIP, Paleo, Low Histamine

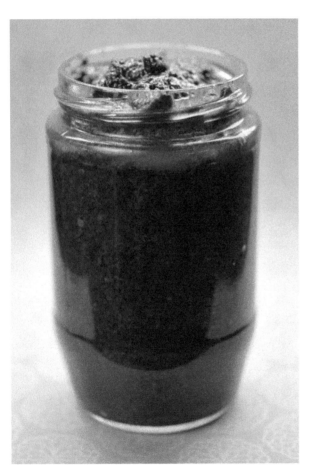

Ingredients:

8 ounces Organic Basil

16 TBSP Organic Extra Virgin Olive Oil

1 1/2 tsp Celtic Sea Salt

3 tsp Organic Dried Minced Onion

1/2 tsp Organic Garlic Powder

pinch of Organic black pepper (Omit for AIP)

Directions:

In a blender, add enough of the oil to cover the blades (be sure to keep a running count of how much oil you're adding). Next, add the basil a bit at time and blend. As you add more basil, add more olive oil, and continue to mix the two together until all of the basil and oil are in the blender. After it's all blended well, add the seasonings and continue to blend to ensure it's well incorporated. A food processor would also work really well in blending your ingredients.

BBQ Sauce

Vegan, Top 8 Free, Free From: Gluten, Coconut, Corn, Legumes, Seeds, Sesame, Sulfites

Ingredients:

12 ounces Organic Tomato Paste

1/2 cup Organic Maple Syrup

1/4 cup Water

2 TBSP Organic Extra Virgin Olive Oil

1/2 TBSP Organic Apple Cider Vinegar

1/4 cup Organic Light Brown Sugar

4 tsp Organic Dried Minced Onion

2 tsp Organic Ground Mustard

1 tsp Celtic Sea Salt

1/2 tsp Organic Garlic Granules

1/2 tsp Organic Cayenne Pepper

Directions:

With a whisk, mix together the tomato paste and wet ingredients. When they're smoothly combined, add in the sugar and seasonings. Continue to whisk until everything is incorporated together. Heat the sauce on low on the stove top. Put a lid on it and let it simmer for 15 – 20 minutes. When doing this, it will thicken up a bit, and become even more yummy.

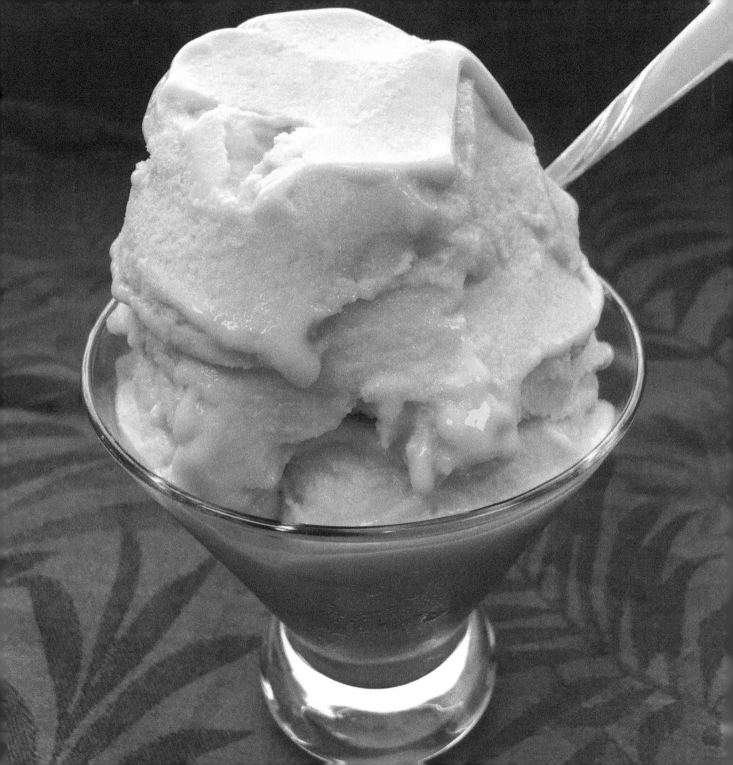

Life is Short... Eat Dessert First

Confession time. It's not uncommon for me to eat a couple of cookies and call it a meal. Why? Because it's safe and easy. With my condition, sometimes that's all I have the energy to deal with, and that's OK. The lesson to learn is that we have to do what's best for us. On the flip side, I do love a good dessert. If you follow us online, you'll know that I have a bit of an obsession with cookies and ice cream. Oh sweet delicious ice cream...

When first diagnosed with food allergies, food intolerances, or starting a new restricted/special/medical diet, I often tell people to do three things. First, feel sorry for yourself. Like, reaaalllyyyy sorry for yourself. In our western world, food is everywhere and part of most major functions and events. You've been handed what can feel like a death sentence. Next, go eat something sweet, even it's as simple as a date. Don't allow yourself to "feel" restricted. If you're more of a savory person, you may want something else. Finally, get busy finding solutions. If all we do is feel sorry for ourselves and complain, nothing will ever get done. So that is exactly why I'm a HUGE fan of dessert. Ice cream is my jam, and I will not let this condition stop me from having some, and neither should you. Want ice cream for breakfast? Go for it. Don't let conventional ideas of meals stop you from what you want and need. Given how limited we already are, I figure, we deserve the treat (picture a winky emoji here).

Tiger Nut Ice Cream

Vegan, Top 8 Free, Free From: Gluten, Cane Sugar, Coconut, Corn, Legumes, Mustard, Nightshades, Seeds, Sesame, Sulfites

Friendly To: Paleo, Low Histamine

Compatible With: AIP

For AIP: Omit xanthan. Your ice cream will be a little more soft-serve, but still delicious.

These are fun and festive during the summer. The fruit can be substituted for whatever you're in the mood for. If you ever make Flag Cake, this would be a great addition to your cake.

Ingredients:

2 cups Tiger Nut Milk

4 - 6 ounces Organic Maple Syrup

1 1/2 tsp Organic Vanilla Extract

1/2 tsp Sea Salt

2 tsp Xanthan (Authentic Foods, Cabbage Derived)

Directions:

Start by adding all of your ingredients to your blender. Blend on high until smooth. Transfer to your ice cream machine and let it do the rest of the work.

If you don't have an ice cream machine, there are other options such as the rock salt method, and the no-churn freezer method.

If you prefer to skip the xanthan, you can also use guar gum, arrowroot, kuzu, tapioca, or potato starches.

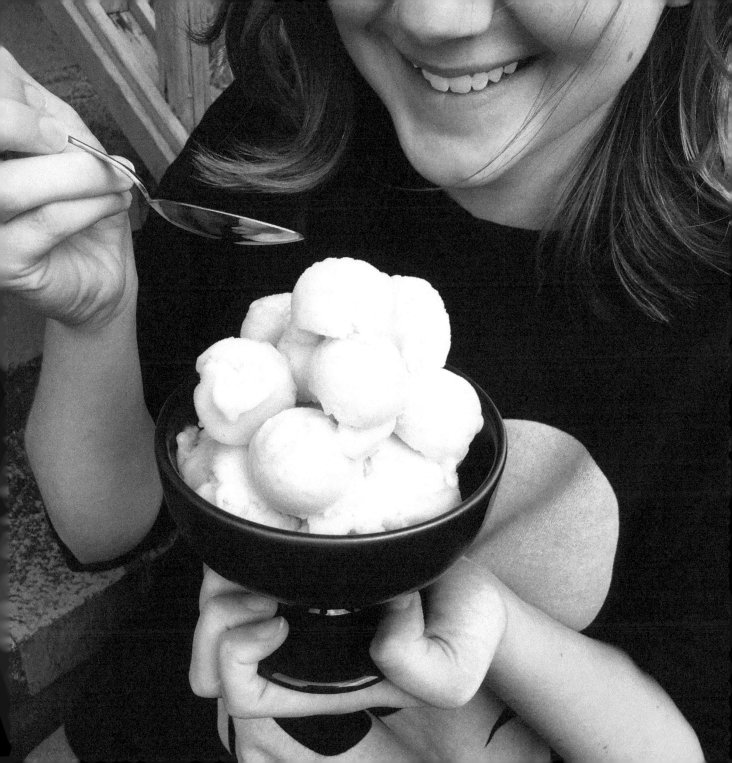

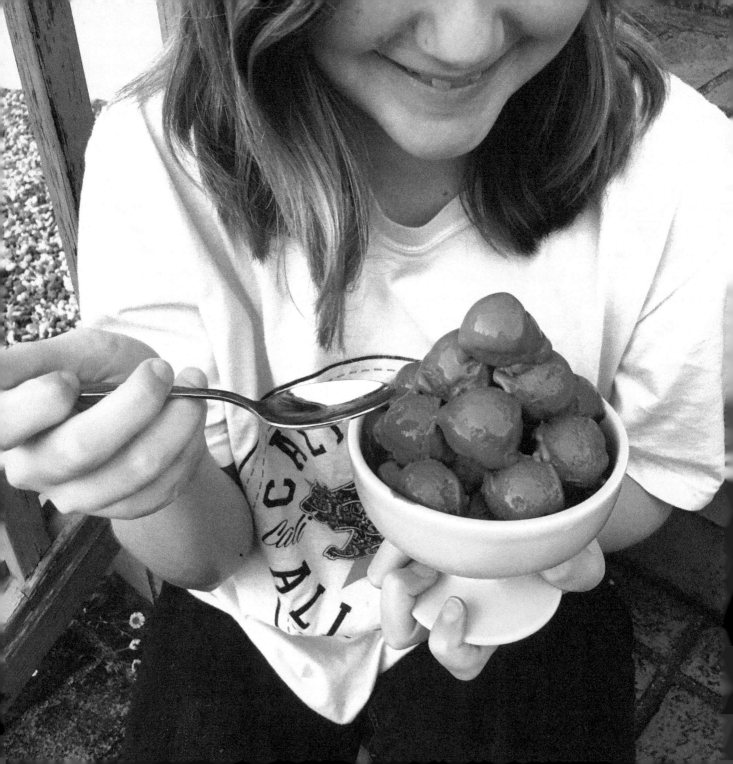

Chocolate Oat Ice Cream

Vegan, Top 8 Free, Free From: Gluten, Coconut, Corn, Legumes, Mustard, Nightshades, Seeds, Sesame, Sulfites

If you love ice cream like we do, this is sure to be a winner in your home. It's also a great ratio for those of you that can tolerate cane sugar and oats. Other tasty flavors we've made: strawberry, vanilla, mint chip, lemon, and more.

Ingredients:

2 cups Oat Milk

100g Dark Brown Sugar

30g Organic Cacao

2 tsp Organic Vanilla Extract

1 tsp Xanthan (Authentic Foods, Cabbage Derived)

1/2 tsp Celtic Sea Salt

Directions:

Start by adding all of your ingredients to your blender. Blend on high until smooth. Transfer to your ice cream machine and let it do the rest of the work.

If you don't have an ice cream machine, there are other options such as the rock salt method, and the no-churn freezer method.

If you prefer to skip the xanthan, you can also use guar gum, arrowroot, kuzu, tapioca, or potato starches.

Sunflower Chocolate Chip Cookies

Vegan, Top 8 Free, Free From: Gluten, Cane Sugar, Corn, Coconut, Legumes, Nightshades, Sesame, Sulfites, Yeast

Friendly To: Diabetic, Paleo

Compatible With: Low Histamine

For Low Histamine: Omit chocolate chips.

These cookies are simply little bites of joy. Take this advice however: make small batches. If you don't, you'll gain 10 pounds. Yes, they're that tasty.

Ingredients:

3.5 ounces Organic Sunflower Seed Butter

4 TBSP Organic Tiger Nut Flour

3 TBSP Cassava Flour

6 tsp Organic Maple Butter

2 TBSP Chocolate Chips

1 TBSP Water

1/4 tsp Sea Salt

Directions:

Combine all of your ingredients together in a bowl. These mix easily by hand, or you can use a stand mixer with the paddle attachment. Next, form dough balls and place them on a baking tray lined with parchment. IMPORTANT: you will need to restrain yourself from eating all of the dough balls as you prep the cookies for baking. Finally, bake at 325 for 13 minutes.

One final friendly tip: Don't burn your mouth trying to eat them when they come out of the oven. I know... life is rough. I truly hope you ENJOY these cookies!

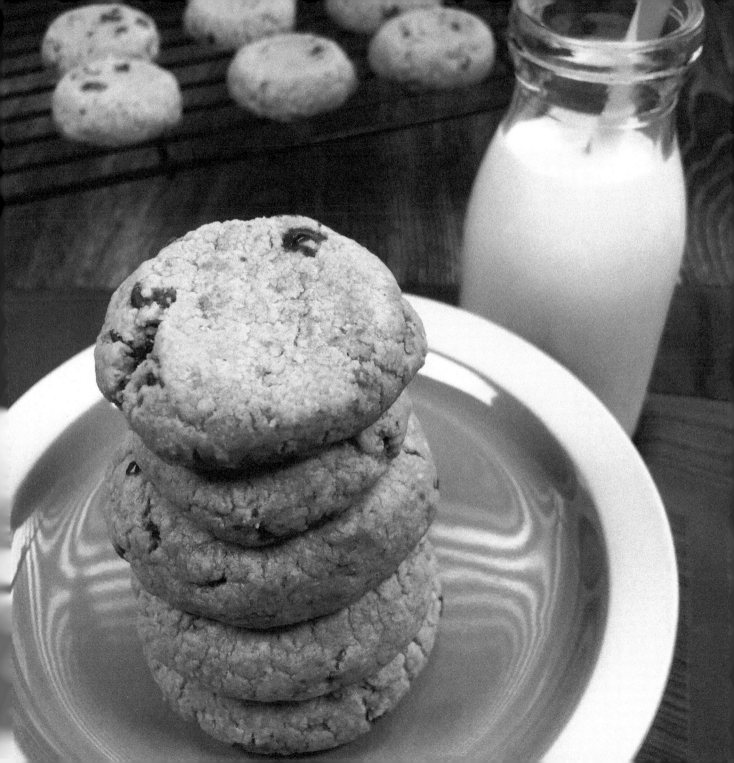

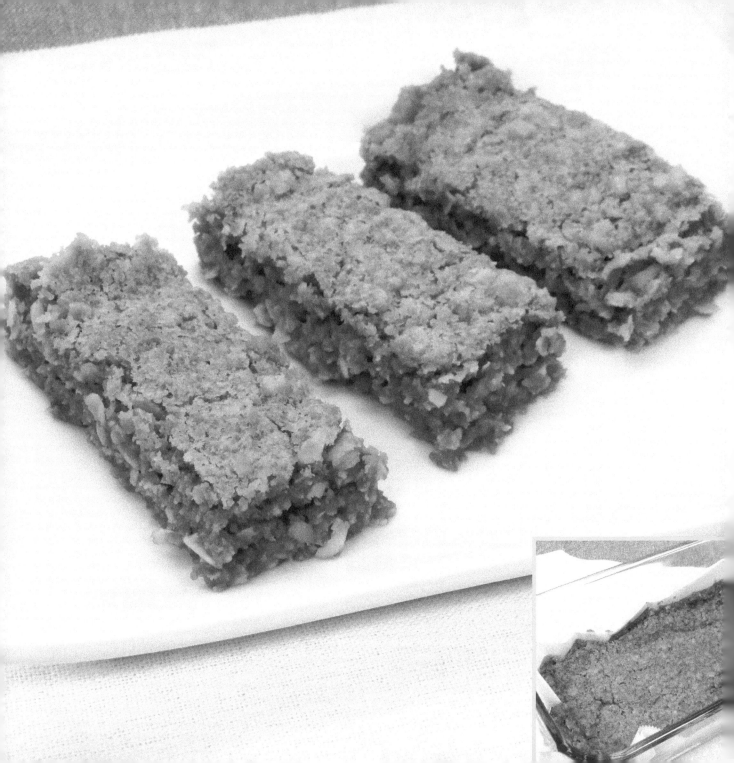

Salted Oat Cookie Loaf

Vegan, Top 8 Free, Free From: Gluten, Coconut, Corn, Legumes, Mustard, Nightshades, Seeds, Sesame, Sulfites

Friendly To: Low Histamine

This cookie loaf is simply delicious. Be sure to look at the Cookie Brittle on the next page too.

Ingredients:

2 cups GF Rolled Oats

300g Dark Brown Sugar, packed (1.5 cups)

140g GF Oat Flour (1 cup)

6 ounces Shortening

4 TBSP Safe Water

1 TBSP Organic Vanilla Extract

1 tsp Celtic Sea Salt

Optional: Pascha Chocolate Chips

Directions:

Place you shortening and sugar in your stand mixer and cream together using the paddle attachment. Scrape down the edges of the bowl and mix again. Next, add in all of the other ingredients, except the water. Pulse, then mix together. Add your water one tablespoon at a time until a dough forms. Transfer your dough to a loaf pan lined with parchment paper.

For Cookie Brittle (see next page) bake for 12 minutes at 325. For Cookie Loaf, bake for 25 minutes at 325.

Behind The Scenes

Can I tell you the problem with the internet, and most blog websites? They often times won't share the failures with you. It leaves readers with the idea of a very perfect kitchen. While we don't have failures in our kitchen too often, when we do, I will look at all of the angles and figure out was it an issue with flavor, texture, technique, or a combination. In the case of what's pictured (we're totally calling it Cookie Brittle), it was amazing in flavor. One could look at these and think fail, however, one would be wrong to do so. As it turns out, if you leave this to cool, it can be picked up. It's crunchier than a standard cookie, and packs in sweetness and flavor. It truly is a Cookie Brittle.

I share this with you because on your journey, not everything is going to work out as you intended, and that's OK, and to be expected. Cooking and baking free-from is no easy task, but once you have the hang of it, there will be no stopping you.

To make Cookie Brittle, we used the recipe on the previous page. Using a medium cookie dough scooper, the dough was portioned and rolled like a traditional cookie. When baked, it spread as pictured. Allow the Cookie Brittle to cool on the tray, and then enjoy. You can also eat it hot :)

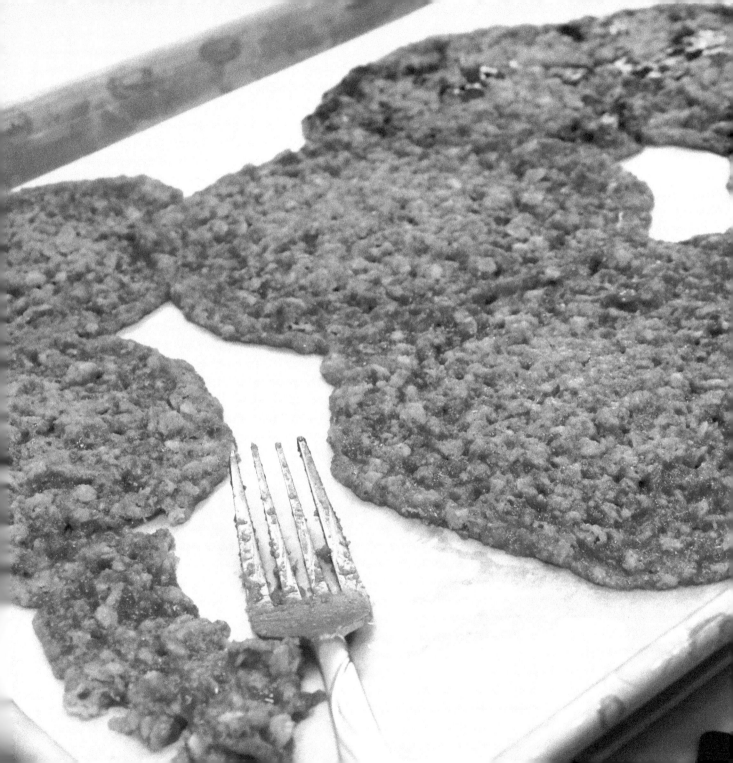

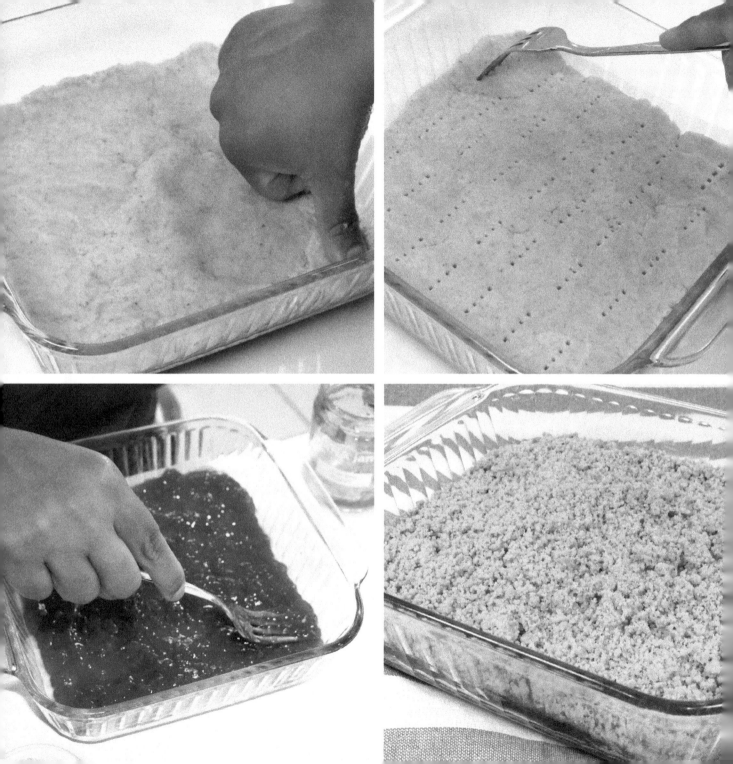

Around Here, We Be Jammin'

There are SO many issues that you will run into when living with a corn allergy, especially a severe one. Jams and jellies are pretty much off the menu, unless you make them yourself. Enter Inna Jam. Now, I'm going to let you know up front, it's about $12 a jar. While it's a lot (the average price of organic jam is $3.50), it's worth every single penny. Inna makes several flavors that are corn free. I can personally vouch for the Peach, Nectarine, and Plout flavors. When placing an order, call and ask to speak with Dafna. You'll need to let her know that you need a batch that's been made with fruit from Ferrari Farm. Tell her The Allergy Chef sent you, and you have a corn allergy.

Inna is nothing short of amazing. It goes well on just about everything I've put it on, and of course, straight out of the jar too. Their transparency is awesome, and dedication to quality is superb.

I know some of you reading don't have a corn allergy. Our favorite top 8 allergy free jam company is Crofters Organic. Hands down, we love them to bits. They even have a line that's free from added sugar. The facility is top 8 free, and it's family owned and operated. They're some of the kindest folks I've ever met, and they have a real desire to help the food allergy and special diet community.

Finally, this recipe can be made with any jam of your choosing.

Jam Crumble

Vegan, Top 8 Free, Free From: Gluten, Cane Sugar, Coconut, Corn, Legumes, Mustard, Nightshades, Sesame, Sulfites
Friendly To: Paleo

For those of you who can't have Inna Jam due to cane sugar, you can make something easy and delicious too. Start with a fruit of your choosing, such as strawberries. Blend with maple (or other safe sweetener). Fold in chia seeds and allow it to set for 20 minutes. Done!

Ingredients:

250g Cassava

125g Shortening

60g Organic Maple Sugar

40g Tiger Nut Flour

2 TBSP Flax + 6 TBSP Safe Water

2 TBSP Safe Oil

2 tsp Organic Vanilla

2 tsp Organic Apple Cider Vinegar

1/2 tsp Baking Soda

Additional Crumble Ingredients:

25g Cassava Flour

25g Tiger Nut Flour

10 ounces Jam of Choice

Directions:

Start by combining your flax and water together and allow it to gel. This takes several minutes. Next, combine the dough ingredients (including your flax gel) together in your food processor. Line a 9x9 baking dish with parchment. Remove 300 grams of dough from your food processor and transfer it to your baking dish. Press it flat, as evenly as possible. Use a fork to poke holes (score) your dough. Next, spread your jam layer evenly across the dough (feel free to use more than 10 oz).

Add the 25 grams of cassava and tiger nut (crumble ingredients) to the dough that's still in your food processor. Pulse everything together, and a very crumbly dough should form. Spread this on top of your jam layer.

Bake at 325 for 20 minutes, uncovered.

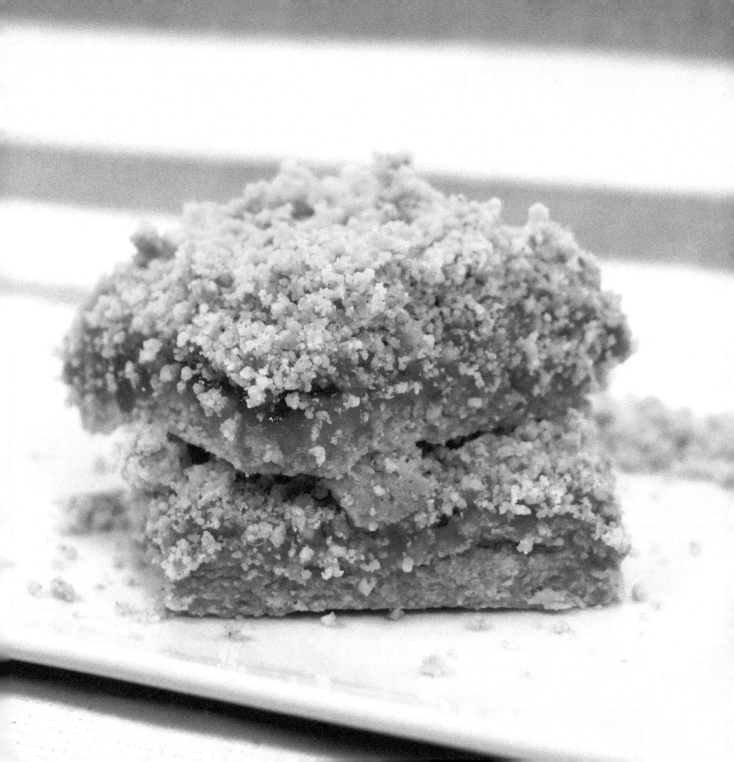

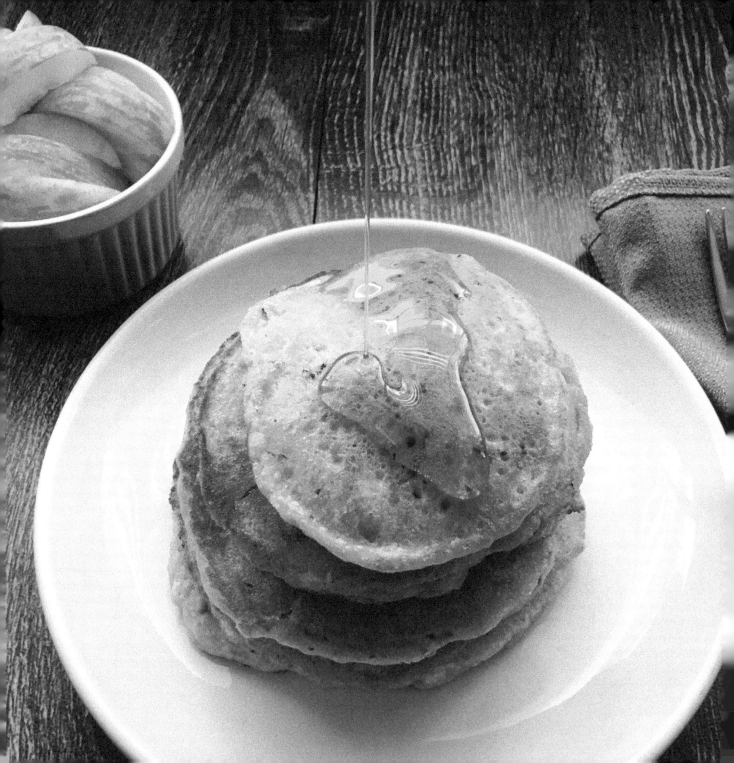

Breakfast Time

As it turns out, there are LOADS of breakfast foods you still have access to, even when living gluten free, corn free, and/or top 8 free. Let's start with the obvious: oatmeal (thank you glutenfreeoats.com), toast (homemade bread of course), pancakes, waffles, bacon, sausage (homemade), smoothies, and juice. Then there's the less obvious: avocado and toast, ice cream, breakfast cookies, fruit with homemade yogurt, overnight oats, chia pudding (fruity variety or chocolate variety), leftover dinner, breakfast pizza, and more.

The real key is figuring out what you like, and from there, creating the individual elements to make it happen. Let's look at overnight oats. For me, that would be safe oats from glutenfreeoats.com, safe water, safe salt, and a safe sweetener. I personally can't have chocolate, so I'll leave that to the rest of you. I can't have oats either, which is why this was a hypothetical meal :) Breakfast pizza looks the same. Safe flour, yeast, water, and oil to form the dough. Safe milk and flour to form the cream sauce. Safe bison and maple for a nice play on sausage. Make a ton and freeze the extras. See! Easy, right? OK, maybe not as easy as ready-made meals, but, it can be done.

Grain Free Waffle

Vegan, Top 8 Free, Free From: Gluten, Cane Sugar, Coconut, Corn, Legumes, Mustard, Nightshades, Sesame, Sulfites

Friendly To: AIP, Paleo

For AIP: Omit the flax and water combo. Your waffles will be more delicate, but still delicious.

After we had our NutraMilk machine, it was like the heavens had opened up and poured ideas down on me. Now that super safe milk was on the menu, so were waffles!! If you're familiar with cassava, you'll know it's a little gummy. Don't let that stop you from enjoying thees. If you're able to have a wide range of pseudo-grains, use 200 grams of your favorite blend.

Ingredients:

200g Cassava Flour

50g Organic Maple Sugar

1 1/4 cup Milk of Choice (we used Tiger Nut Milk)

3 TBSP Flax + 6 TBSP Safe Water

4 TBSP Safe Oil

3 tsp Organic Apple Cider Vinegar

1/2 tsp Baking Soda

1/2 tsp Celtic Sea Salt

Directions:

Start by combining your flax and water. It will take several minutes for them to gel together. Next, measure out your milk, and add the apple cider vinegar to the milk. Next, combine all of your dry ingredients together in your stand mixer, and mix using the wire attachment. Add the milk/acv mix and pulse together. You'll see the acv and baking soda react. Allow your mix to sit for a minute untouched. Finally, add in the rest of the wet ingredients and mix well.

Using your waffle maker with your preferred settings, make waffles. A note about the texture: cassava waffles are a bit on the gummy side, even when well cooked. It can take some getting use to, but is quite delicious.

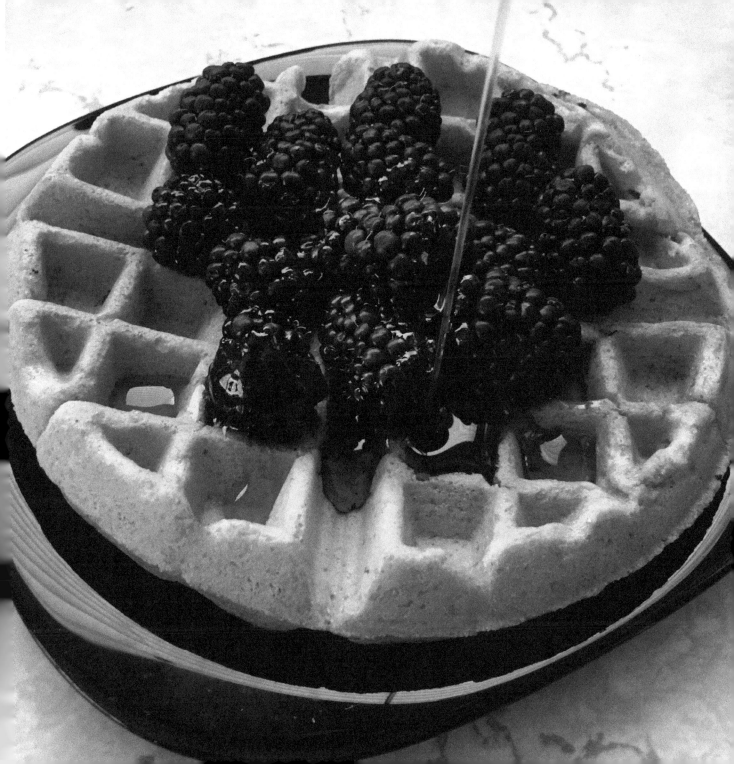

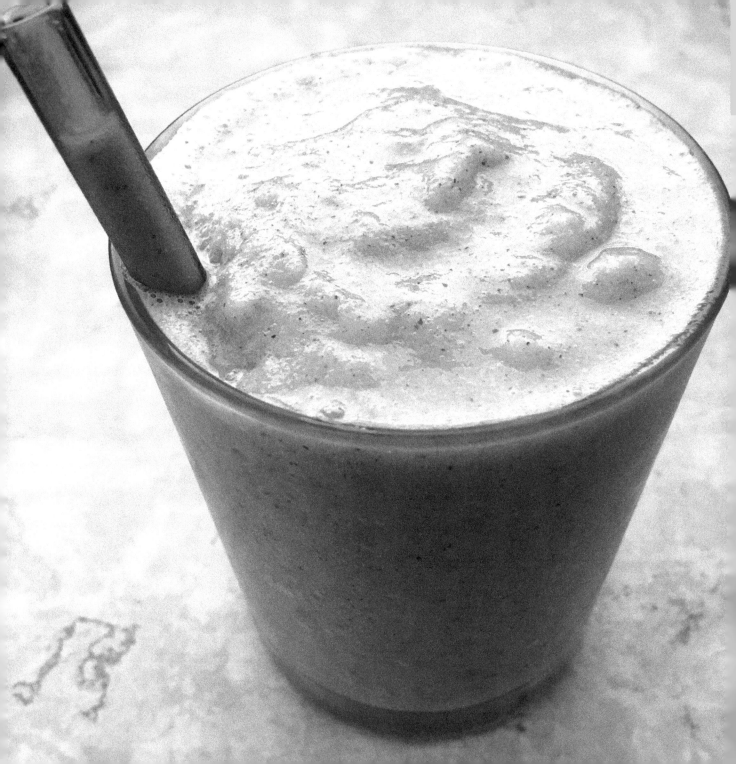

Green Shake Smoothie

Vegan, Top 8 Free, Free From: Gluten, Cane Sugar, Coconut, Corn, Legumes, Mustard, Nightshades, Seeds, Sesame, Sulfites

Friendly To: AIP, Paleo, Low Histamine

Bananas are a cornerstone of the smoothie world. So what about those of us with a corn allergy? How do we go about thickening our smoothies??? The answer is so unconventional: frozen veggies. Zucchini has a very mellow flavor, and you won't notice it too much. Yet, you'll love it because it won't water down your drink like ice would have.

Ingredients:

1 cup Tiger Nut Milk

Frozen Safe Zucchini

Safe Maple Syrup

Directions:

Pour your milk into your blender. Next, add your preferred amount of frozen zucchini and maple syrup and blend. I like to add enough zucchini to have a milkshake texture, rather than a thick smoothie texture. I also like it to taste like a milkshake, so I don't skimp on the maple syrup.

Additionally, you can add other safe (frozen) fruits to change the flavor profile of your drink. I've experimented with grapes, tangerines, and blackberries.

Cinnamon Oat Pancakes

Vegan, Top 8 Free, Free From: Gluten, Cane Sugar, Coconut, Corn, Legumes, Mustard, Sesame, Sulfites

The oats in this recipe add an extra depth of flavor. It's also a recipe that's free from cane sugar, making it a favorite in our house. Be sure to compare this to the recipe on page 70 for more pancake goodness.

Ingredients:

1.5 cup Organic Oat Flour

1 cup Sorghum Flour, superfine

2/3 cup Organic Maple Sugar

4 TBSP Arrowroot

3 TBSP Golden Flax

4 tsp Baking Powder

4 tsp Organic Ground Cinnamon

1/2 tsp Sea Salt

8 ounces Milk of Choice

4 tsp Raw Organic Apple Cider Vinegar

Directions:

Combine your milk and apple cider vinegar together and set aside. Next, add all of your other ingredients together in your stand mixer and mix using the wire attachment. Add in the milk and mix well until your batter is smooth and there are no lumps.

We like to make pancakes on medium heat in a safe, non-stick pan.

These pancakes have been topped with Inna Peach Jam, and served with pomegranate seeds from a safe farm in our area.

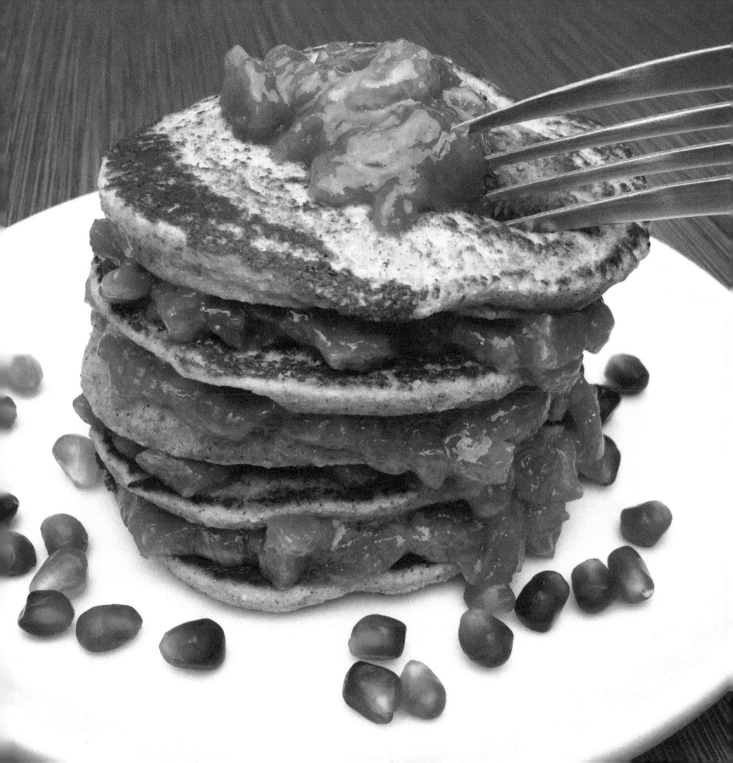

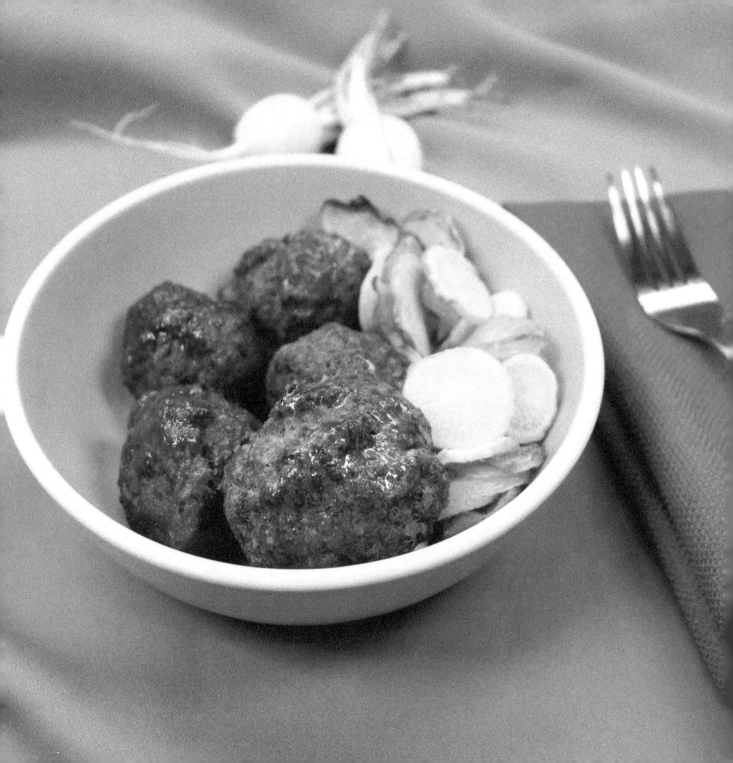

Bacon Bison Meatballs

Top 8 Free, Free From: Gluten, Cane Sugar, Coconut, Corn, Legumes, Mustard, Nightshades, Seeds, Sesame, Sulfites

Friendly To: AIP, Paleo

These meatballs are nothing short of amazing. It all starts with safe bison from The Honest Bison. We pair it with safe, local, bacon. The bacon that we source only has a few added spices, including thyme and salt. If you don't have bacon available to you, see about sourcing safe pork belly, and make your own. You'll notice this recipe doesn't call for many ingredients, and that's because the bacon is so flavorful. Another alternative if you can't find safe bacon is to use a safe cut of pork and grind it at home. Add your desired spices and blend with your bison.

Ingredients:

1 pound Ground Bison

.7 lb Safe Bacon

1 1/2 tsp Organic Oregano

Directions:

In your food processor, combine your bison, bacon, and oregano. Mix until very well combined. Portion your meat into 12 jumbo meatballs and bake at 425 for 20 minutes.

Why no salt? It's all in the bacon. We have a local provider of safe bacon that only uses three ingredients on the bacon. It's not smoked and it's uncured. Selecting safe bacon will be the challenge for this recipe, but it is possible. Both EatWild and LocalHarvest are websites that can help you connect with farmers in your area, or those who may be willing to ship.

These meatballs have been served with local, safe, turnips that were roasted in safe olive oil.

Cinnamon Pancakes

Vegan, Top 8 Free, Free From: Gluten, Cane Sugar, Coconut, Corn, Legumes, Mustard, Seeds, Sesame, Sulfites

Friendly To: AIP, Paleo

This pancake recipe is a great go-to for basic ratios. If you're not in the mood for cinnamon, what about lemon? Or chocolate? Maybe even add in some Pascha Chocolate Chips. There are so many safe options for you to explore once you get the ratios down. Happy pancaking!!

Ingredients:

150g Sorghum Flour, superfine

150g Millet Flour, superfine

80g Organic Dark Brown Sugar

40g Arrowroot

2 cups Milk of Choice

4 TBSP Flax + 8 TBSP Safe Water

3 TBSP Safe Oil

4 tsp Baking Powder

4 tsp Organic Cinnamon

1 TBSP Apple Cider Vinegar

2 tsp Organic Vanilla Extract

1/2 tsp Celtic Sea Salt

Directions:

Start by combining your flax and water. It will take several minutes for them to gel together. Next, measure out your milk, and add the apple cider vinegar to the milk. Next, combine all of your dry ingredients together in your stand mixer, and mix using the wire attachment. Add the milk/acv mix and pulse together. You'll see the acv and baking soda react. Allow your mix to sit for a minute untouched. Finally, add in the rest of the wet ingredients and mix well.

We like to make pancakes on medium heat in a safe, non-stick pan.

These pancakes have been served with tiger nut milk, local safe fruit, and local safe bacon.

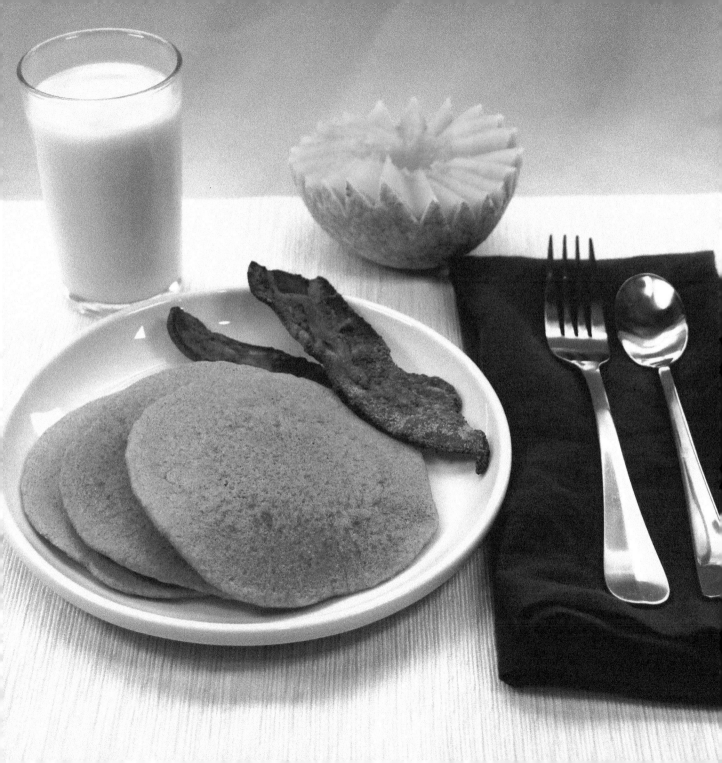

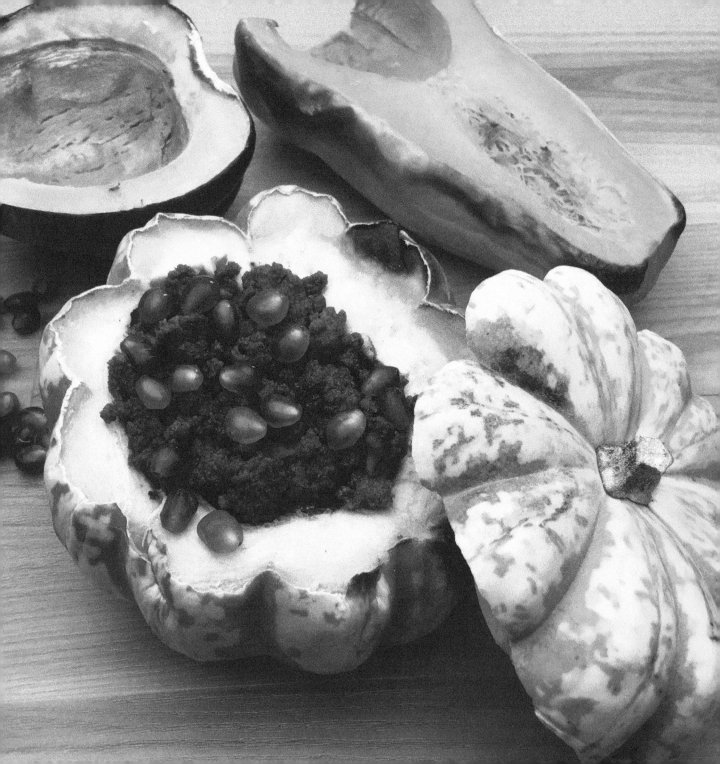

Lunch & Dinner

Some say lunch is the hardest meal of the day for those who are living with multiple and severe food allergies. The part most people find difficult is creating/finding meals that are good for on-the-go, and taste good hot or cold. Personally, leftovers are what we turn to many for lunches. Other times, since the kids are home-schooled, hot lunches are created. It's not uncommon for me to make extra staples such as cooked rice or caramelized onions for random use throughout the week. It's something you'll need to get use to.

For those of you who live a very busy life outside of the home, you'll want to have at least one meal prep day a week. This way, there's a huge stressor removed from your working days. For those of you who are corn free, use glass containers when possible, and be picky about lids. Many commercially available plastic lids contain corn derivatives.

Finally, when creating food that you enjoy, make double or triple batches and freeze the extras in lunch-sized containers. You'll find that as your freezer stock grows, the daily struggle seems to melt away. Oh, and don't forget to pack cookies in your lunch :) For more lunch ideas and recipes, be sure to check out our cookbook: The Gluten Free Allergy Friendly Lunch Box.

Let's Talk About Yeast

I'll be the first to admit it: working with yeast can seem intimidating. The first time we worked with it, our creation was a total failure. It took me a long time to muster up the courage to try again (that and we were super busy with life). A very good friend of ours offered to video chat me through the process since they were a yeast master. Having someone guide me that second time was all I needed. Since then, I've been off making all sorts of fun foods with yeast. Here are some tips I want to pass on to you:

- Sites such as youtube may offer you a video tutorial which can be beneficial.
- If you have a good food thermometer, use it.
- I personally bring my water and sweetener to a boil, then remove it from the heat. As it cools, I check on it every couple of minutes. When I can dip in a finger without being burned, but also not luke-warm, I add the yeast.
- I like to gently mix the yeast in with a fork before it activates.

Pictured is what your yeast should look like if it has activated successfully.

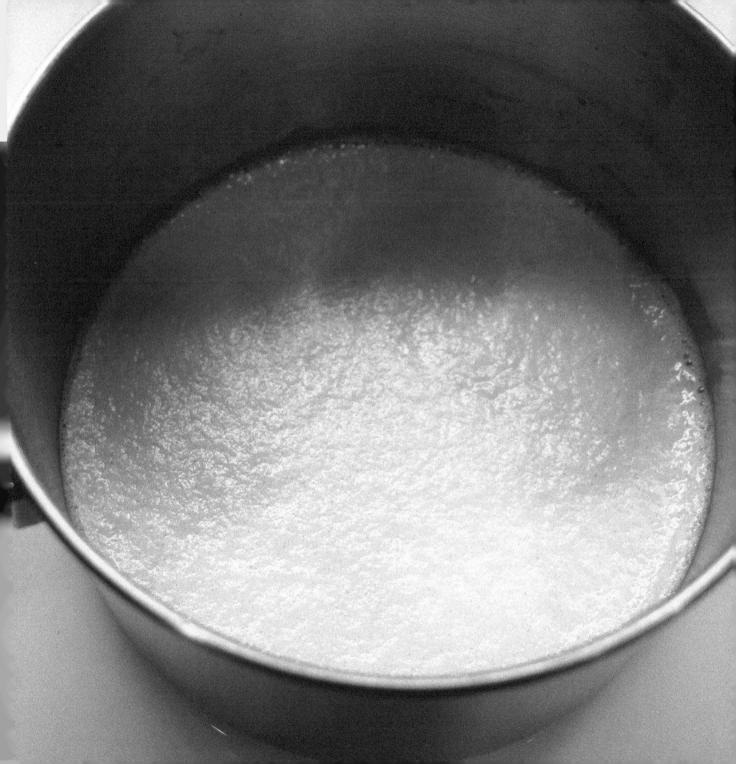

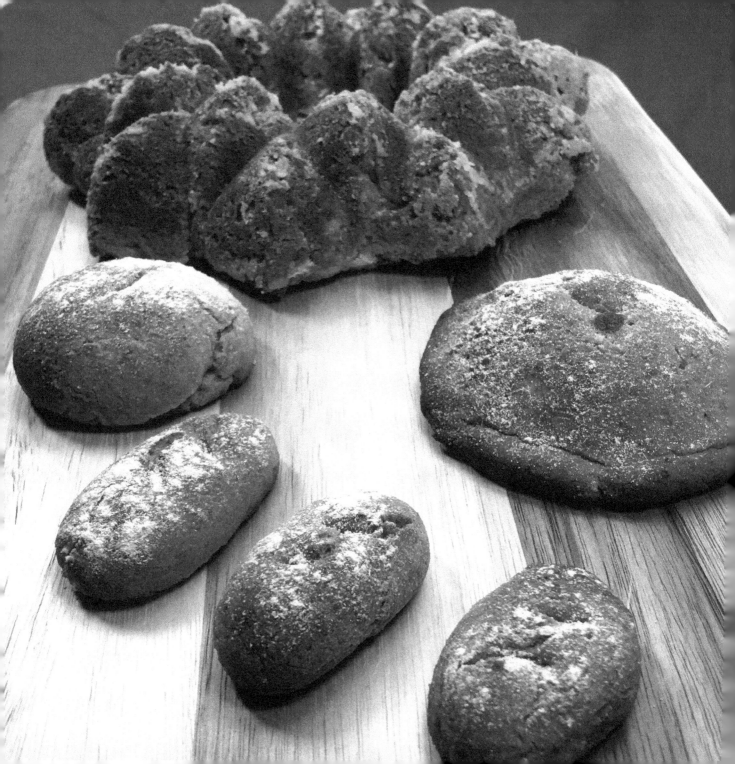

Bread – Sweet, Sweet, Bread

Vegan, Top 8 Free, Free From: Gluten, Cane Sugar, Coconut, Corn, Legumes, Mustard, Nightshades, Seeds, Sesame, Sulfites

Friendly To: Paleo

This recipe has been adapted from Otto's Naturals.

Ingredients:

Yeast Mix:

8 ounces Safe Water

4 ounces Maple Syrup

2 Red Star Yeast Packets

Bread Ingredients:

2 cups Cassava Flour

2 tsp Celtic Sea Salt

5 TBSP Flax + 10 TBSP Safe Water

5 TBSP Organic Tiger Nut Oil

3 ounces Organic Maple Syrup

2 ounces Water

Tasty Tip:

This bread is a fantastic base for hand pies. Pictured (large circles in the middle) are bread rolls that have been stuffed with creamy ground meat and seasonings.

Directions:

First, heat your water and maple syrup together, then add the yeast packets. Allow the yeast to activate for 5 - 10 minutes. Next, combine your flax and water to allow it to gel together.

For this recipe, you can mix by hand, or use a stand mixer. I prefer to mix by hand. Combine the bread ingredients, flax gel, and yeast mix together and mix until a dough forms. Cover your bowl with a warm damp paper-towel and allow it to rise for 30 - 60 minutes.

If you're making a loaf, a bundt pan works best. Coat it with oil and flour, then add your dough. Score your dough, then sprinkle additional flour on top.

If you're making bite-sized breads, bake dough balls on parchment paper. You will still want to put oil and flour on your parchment, and sprinkle additional flour on top of your dough balls. This is all done to prevent burning.

Bake at 400 for 30 minutes in a bundt pan, or for 21 minutes as bite-sized bread rolls.

Garlic Knots

Vegan, Top 8 Free, Free From: Gluten, Cane Sugar, Coconut, Corn, Legumes, Mustard, Nightshades, Seeds, Sesame, Sulfites

Friendly To: Paleo

Ingredients:

Yeast Mix:

8 ounces Safe Water

4 ounces Maple Syrup

2 Red Star Yeast Packets

Bread Ingredients:

2 cups Cassava Flour

3 tsp Celtic Sea Salt

5 TBSP Flax + 10 TBSP Safe Water

5 TBSP Avocado Oil

1/3 cup Safe Water

Fresh Chopped Garlic

Organic Parsley for Garnish

Directions:

Follow the instructions on page 77 using the ingredients listed on this page. For the garlic, chop as many cloves as you'd like, and incorporate it with all of the other ingredients.

This dough is much more sticky than the one on page 77, and that's OK. Line a tray with parchment paper, but you won't be using the oil/flour technique this time. Pull out a small handful of dough and roll it out a bit like a hotdog. Manipulate the dough to form what looks like a knot, or mini pretzel. Place it on your tray. Do this until all of the dough has been used. Brush the bread with avocado oil and sprinkle with parsley before baking.

Bake at 350 for 25 minutes. The texture will be a bit on the gummy side when it's fresh from the oven, but will become more bread like as it cools, and much more so the next day. Do not store your bread in the fridge. We've seen the best results from covering the bread with foil, and leaving it on the countertop.

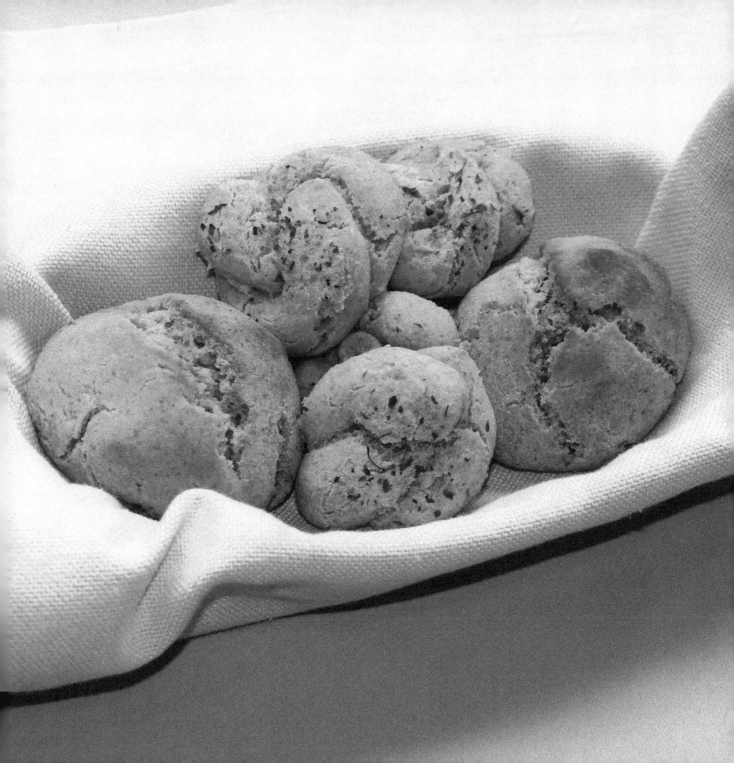

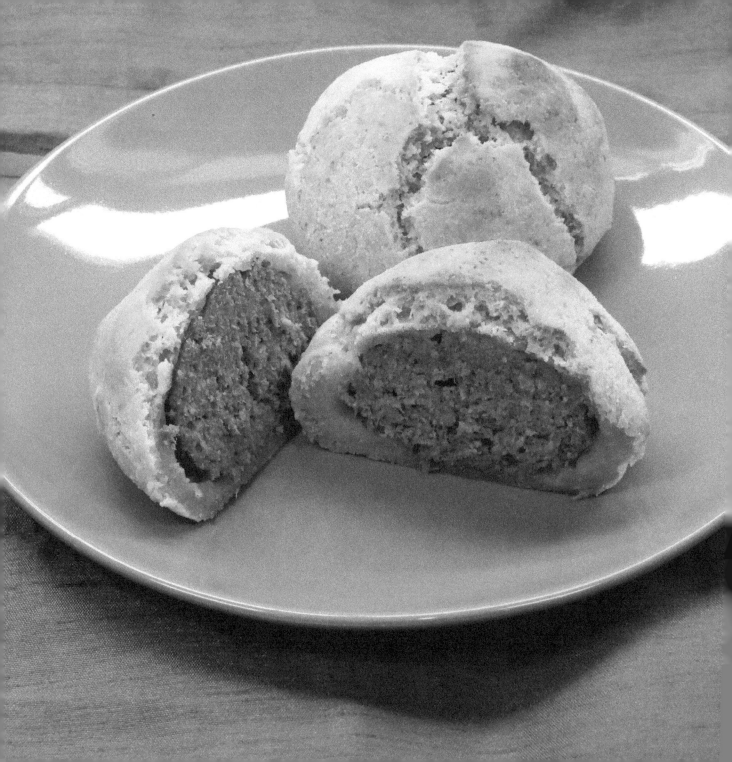

Garlic Meatballs

Vegan, Top 8 Free, Free From: Gluten, Cane Sugar, Coconut, Corn, Legumes, Mustard, Nightshades, Seeds, Sesame, Sulfites

Friendly To: AIP, Paleo

Corn Free: Source safe ingredients. A farmer's market could be particularly helpful with this meal.

Ingredients:

Bacon Bison Meatballs (page 69)

Garlic Knots Dough (page 78)

Directions:

This creation was nothing short of oh my goodness why didn't I make more?! To make these beauties, start with cooked meatballs, and the dough for Garlic Knots.

Take a handful of dough and press it flat. Place a meatball on top and cover completely. Roll the ball in your hands to ensure complete coverage. Bake on a tray lined with parchment paper at 350 for 25 minutes.

Although these are stored in the fridge, they are still so incredibly delicious when eaten cold.

Mini Bison Pockets

Top 8 Free, Free From: Gluten, Cane Sugar, Coconut, Corn, Legumes, Mustard, Nightshades, Seeds, Sesame, Sulfites

Friendly To: Low Histamine

The first time we made these, it was like a party in your mouth... the kind of party that you haven't had for so long because of your diagnosis. The kind of win that we all need, yes, it was one of those meals. Be sure to take these ratios and get to experimenting and creating all sorts of delicious variations.

Ingredients:

Pastry Ingredients:

2 cups Organic Oat Flour

6 TBSP Organic Extra Virgin Olive Oil

3 tsp AIP Paleo Powder

2 tsp Sea Salt

1/2 tsp Garlic Granules

Filling Ingredients:

1 pound Ground Bison

3 TBSP Organic Maple Sugar

2 TBSP Organic Onion Granules

2 tsp Sea Salt

Directions:

In a mixing bowl, combine all of your pastry ingredients together. AIP Paleo Powder is a season blend, and can be purchased online.

In a separate mixing bowl, mix all of your filling ingredients together.

To assemble, take a small handful of pastry and press it flat in your hand. Add filling, then cover completely. We opted to shape ours a bit like rectangles.

Place your pockets on a tray lined with parchment paper and bake at 400 for 16 - 20 minutes.

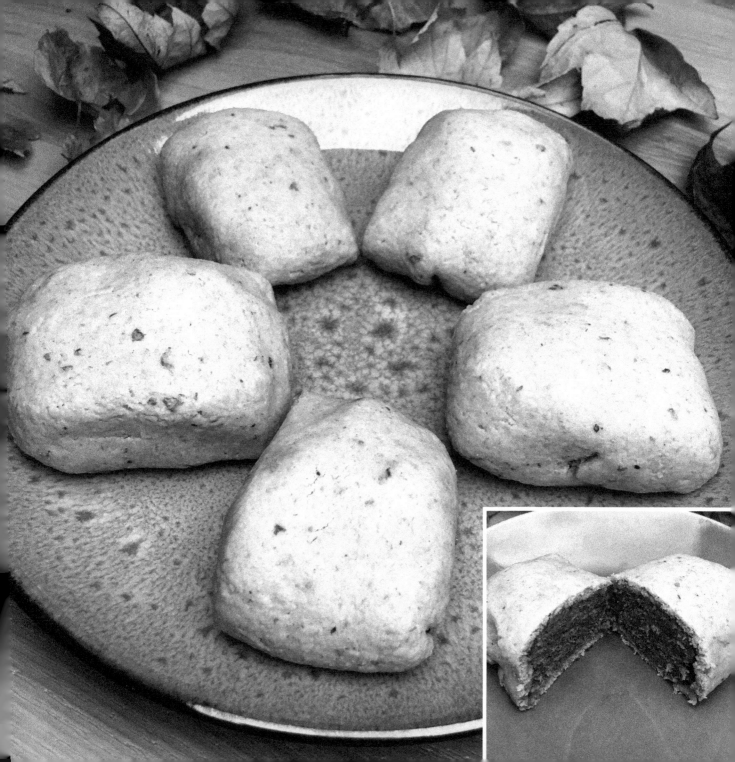

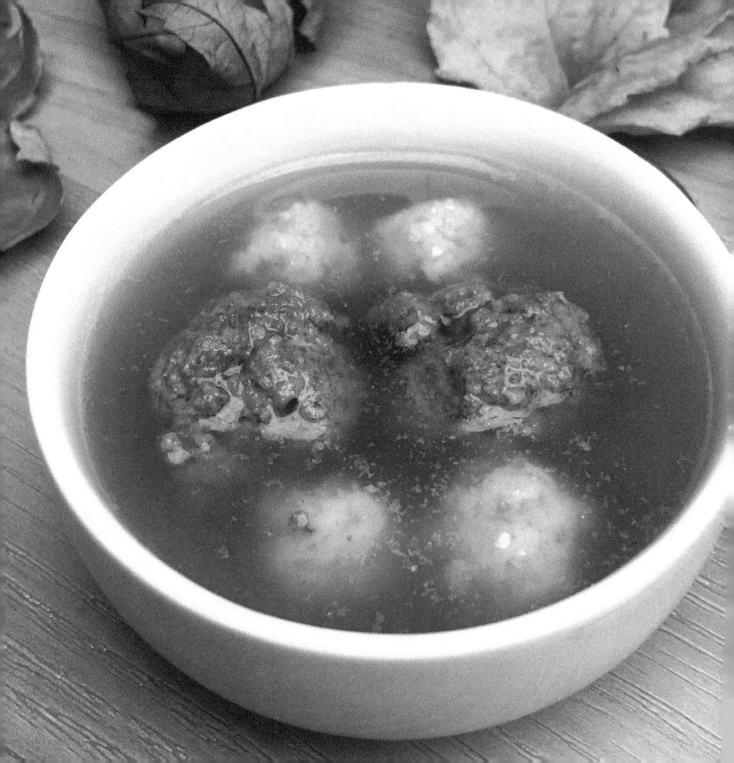

Bison Dumpling Soup

Top 8 Free, Free From: Gluten, Cane Sugar, Coconut, Corn, Legumes, Mustard, Nightshades, Seeds, Sesame, Sulfites

Friendly To: Low Histamine

Compatible With: AIP, Paleo

For AIP & Paleo: Use cassava flour instead of oat flour.

Ingredients:

Dumpling Ingredients:

2 cups Organic Oat Flour

6 TBSP Organic Extra Virgin Olive Oil

3 tsp AIP Paleo Powder

2 tsp Sea Salt

1/2 tsp Garlic Granules

Meatball Ingredients:

1 pound Ground Bison

3 TBSP Organic Maple Sugar

2 TBSP Organic Onion Granules

2 tsp Sea Salt

Directions:

These are the same ingredients as page 82, made in an alternative way. In a mixing bowl, combine all of your pastry ingredients together. In a separate bowl, combine the meatball ingredients together.

Pictured are mini meatballs, made using a small cookie dough scooper (2 tsp). Portion out meatballs and bake on a tray lined with parchment at 400 for 14 - 18 minutes.

Meanwhile, in a stock or stock/water combination of your choosing, bring your liquid to a boil, and add drops of dumpling dough. It cooks quickly. Add your meatballs and serve.

The dumplings are delicate, yet delicious. Pictured is a soup that was made with homemade bone broth.

Pulled BBQ Bison

Top 8 Free, Free From: Gluten, Cane Sugar, Coconut, Corn, Legumes, Mustard, Seeds, Sesame, Sulfites

Friendly To: Paleo

Ingredients:

Shredded Bison:

2.5 pound Inside Round Bison Roast

1 large Yellow Onion, cut into large pieces

1 large Purple Onion, cut into large pieces

32 ounces Safe Water

1 TBSP Apple Cider Vinegar

2 - 3 tsp Celtic Sea Salt

Sauce:

7 ounces Yellow Barn Tomato Concentrate

3 ounces Safe Water

6 tsp YS Honey

3 TBSP Dark Brown Sugar

4 tsp Organic Onion Granules

1 TBSP Apple Cider Vinegar

3/4 tsp Celtic Sea Salt

1/2 tsp Organic Smoked Paprika

pinch Organic Black Pepper

Directions:

Special Tool: Pressure Cooker

Start by rubbing all the sides of your bison with salt. Place it in your pressure cooker, and add the cut onion, vinegar, and water. Gently mix, then cook. We used the meat setting on our pressure cooker for 50 minutes.

For the sauce, combine all of the ingredients together in a small sauce pan on medium heat. Whisk well and allow the sauce to simmer for 15 minutes.

When the meat is done, you will have an abundance, which is exactly what folks like us need. See page 93 for tacos :) To shred the meat, place it on a plate or tray and pull apart with two large forks. For this meal, take a portion of meat and combine with the sauce. Store your extras separate, so you can have different uses for your extra shredded bison.

Pictured along with Garlic Knots and safe carrots.

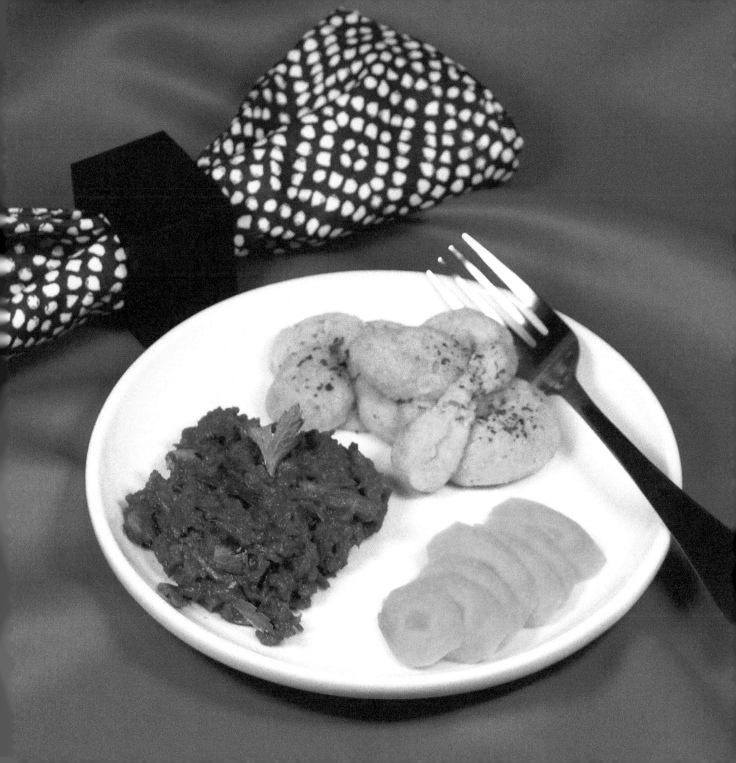

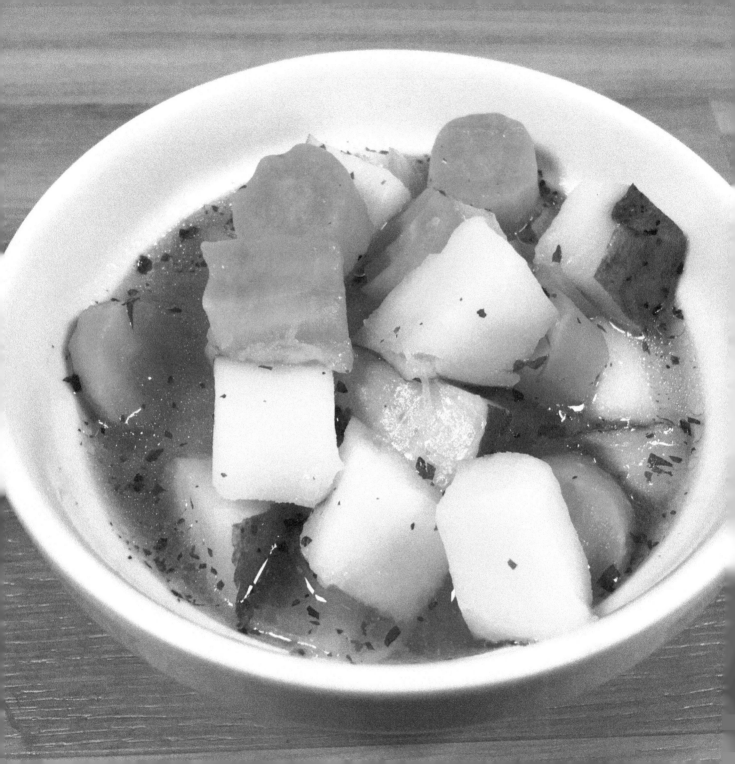

Veggie Soup

Vegan, Top 8 Free, Free From: Gluten, Cane Sugar, Coconut, Corn, Legumes, Mustard, Seeds, Sesame, Sulfites

Friendly To: Low Histamine

Simple, warm, and delicious. Don't let the ease of this meal fool you. During the fall and winter, it will truly hit the spot. This also pairs well with extra shredded bison from page 86.

Ingredients:

2 pounds Organic Potatoes, cubed

1 pound Organic Carrots, medium sized slices

Safe Water

Celtic Sea Salt

Dried Parsley

Directions:

This can be made on the stove top, or in a pressure cooker. It's the type of creation that you'll want to season to taste.

Place your vegetables in a pot and cover with safe water. Bring to a boil, and allow it to boil for several minutes. Turn the heat to medium-low and allow it to simmer until the veggies are fork tender.

If you're using a pressure cooker, add all of your ingredients, and use the appropriate setting. In our case, we would use the soup setting.

Veggie Bison Meatballs

Top 8 Free, Free From: Gluten, Cane Sugar, Coconut, Corn, Legumes, Mustard, Nightshades, Seeds, Sesame, Sulfites

Friendly To: AIP, Paleo, Low Histamine

Paleo: Use olive oil (or oil of choice) instead of butter.
GAPs: Use a legal butter, or olive oil.

Ingredients:

1 pound Bison Blend (6-6-4)

1 medium Carrot (2.5 ounces)

1 medium Zucchini (6 ounces)

1 TBSP Organic Onion Granules

2 tsp Organic Dried Parsley

1 tsp Celtic Sea Salt

3/4 tsp Organic Garlic Granules

Directions:

Start by washing your veggies, and peeling the carrots. Shred the vegetables and place them in a mixing bowl. Add your ground bison and seasonings, and mix well until everything is well incorporated. Pictured are mini meatballs made with 3/4 a scoop of a small cookie dough scooper.

Bake at 425 12 minutes for mini meatballs.

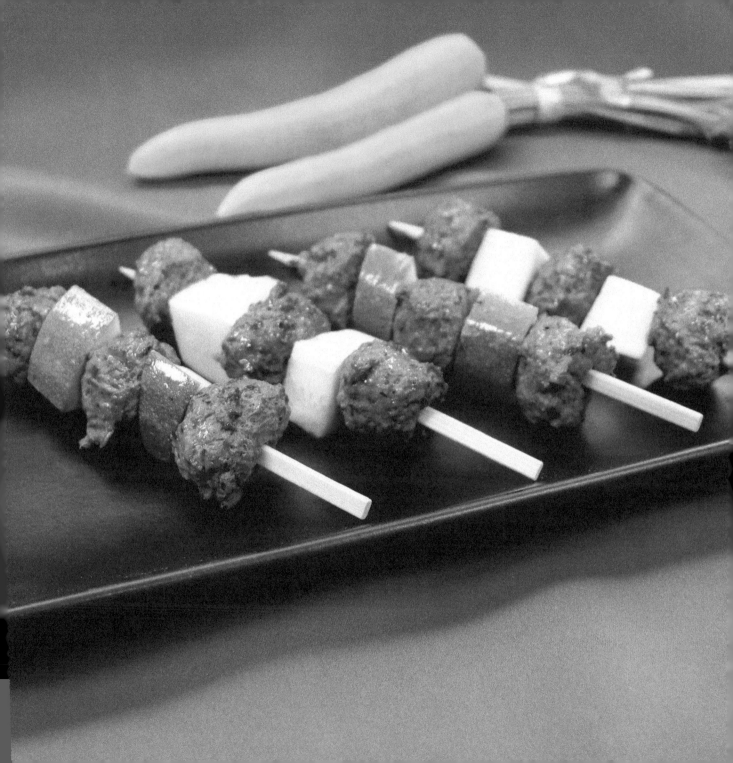

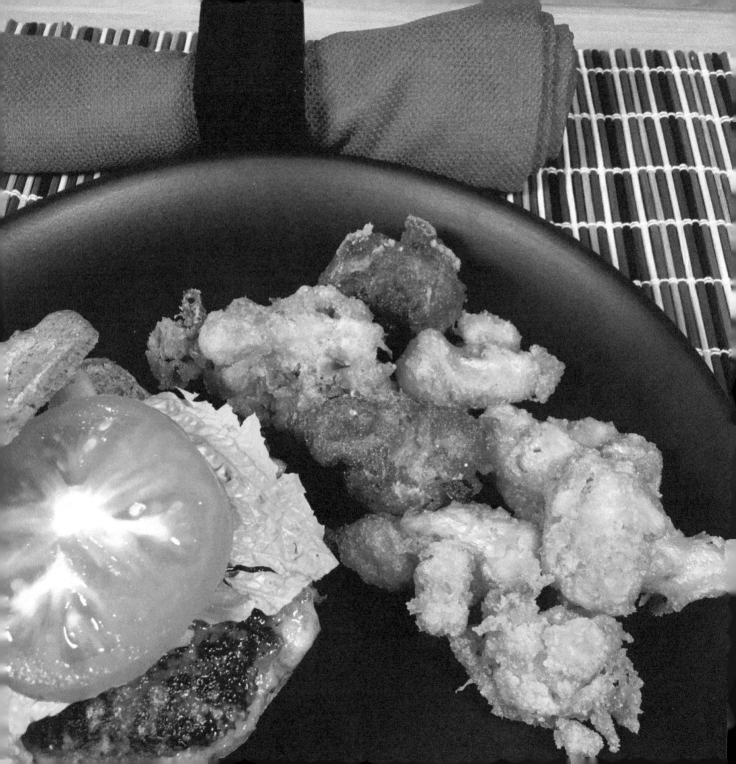

Fried Cauliflower

Vegan, Top 8 Free, Free From: Gluten, Cane Sugar, Coconut, Corn, Legumes, Mustard, Seeds, Sesame, Sulfites

Think you can't have fried food? Think again. There's nothing stopping folks like us from having everything that's delicious, and a real treat. The kids don't love cauliflower standalone... they argued over who received a larger portion of fried cauliflower. For those of you who are corn free, they key is safe ingredient sourcing.

Ingredients:

16 ounces Cauliflower Florets

Safe Oil for Frying

Batter:

140g Millet Flour, superfine

50g Sorghum Flour, superfine

6 ounces Milk of Choice

3 tsp Baking Powder

2 tsp Raw Organic Apple Cider Vinegar

1 tsp Sea Salt

Directions:

Start by pouring your frying oil in a medium or large sized pot and heat on high. Next, break your cauliflower into small and medium sized pieces. Next, combine all of the batter ingredients together in a large mixing bowl. Add your cauliflower heads to the batter and mix well. You want a all of cauliflower to be nicely coated. By now, your oil should be heated and ready for frying. To test, dip a fork in your batter then place the fork in your oil. If it begins to cook right away, you're ready to fry. Using a frying spider, carefully add scoops of your cauliflower to the oil. You may want to use a splatter guard as well. When the cauliflower is golden brown, remove it from the oil and place on paper-towels to soak up excess oil.

For GF and Top 8 Free, canola or avocado oil (or other preferred/safe oil) can be used. For corn free, safe olive oil or tiger nut oil can be used.

Honey Mustard Bacon & Potatoes

Top 8 Free, Free From: Gluten, Cane Sugar, Coconut, Corn, Legumes, Sesame, Sulfites

This is awesome as a breakfast, lunch, or dinner. The bacon adds so much depth, and the flavors help mask the fact that the rice is cauliflower rice (for those of you who may not love cauliflower).

Ingredients:

28 ounces Gold Potatoes (approx 4)

1 pound Safe Bacon, cut into small pieces

1 medium Onion, diced

6 TBSP Honey

2 - 3 TBSP Eden Brown Mustard

For The Rice:

18 ounces Cauliflower Rice

1 tsp Celtic Salt

1/2 tsp Thyme

dashes Ground Ginger

1T honey

Directions:

This meal is all about the prep. Before cooking, you'll want to cut your bacon into small pieces and set aside. Next, use a shredder to rice your cauliflower head. For some, depending on the allergy, you may be able to purchase safe frozen riced cauliflower. Next, cube your potatoes and dice your onion. Now you're ready to start cooking. You'll want to have two pans going at the same time, one for the potatoes and one for the rice.

Heat a large pan and add your bacon, potato cubes, and onion. Cook on medium-high heat for 8 minutes, stirring regularly to prevent burning. Next, add the honey and mustard. Mix well and cover with a lid. Turn the heat to medium-low and cook until the potatoes are easy to pierce with a fork.

For the rice, heat a medium pan and add all of the ingredients on medium heat. Cook for 10 - 12 minutes, stirring regularly. Serve your potatoes over the rice and enjoy.

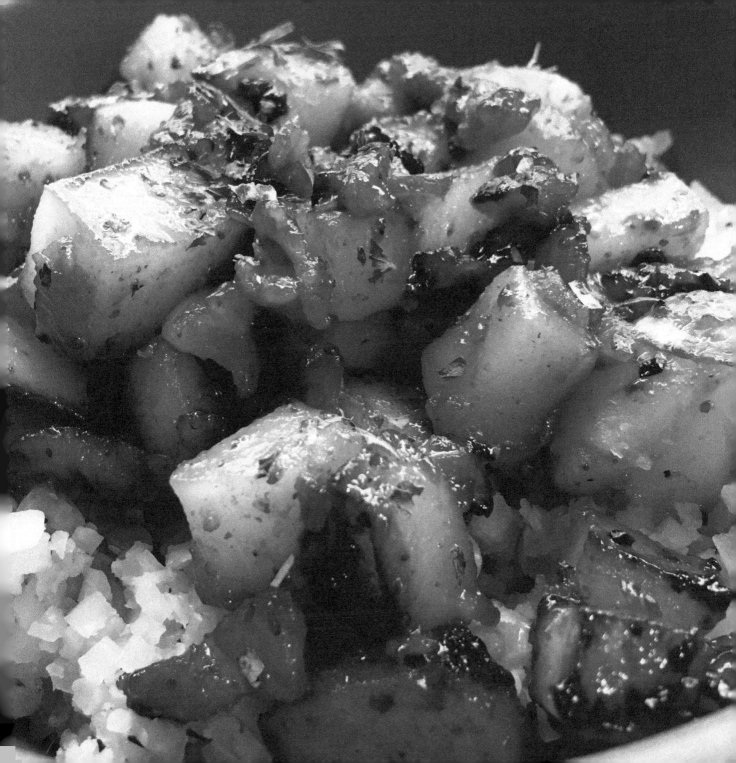

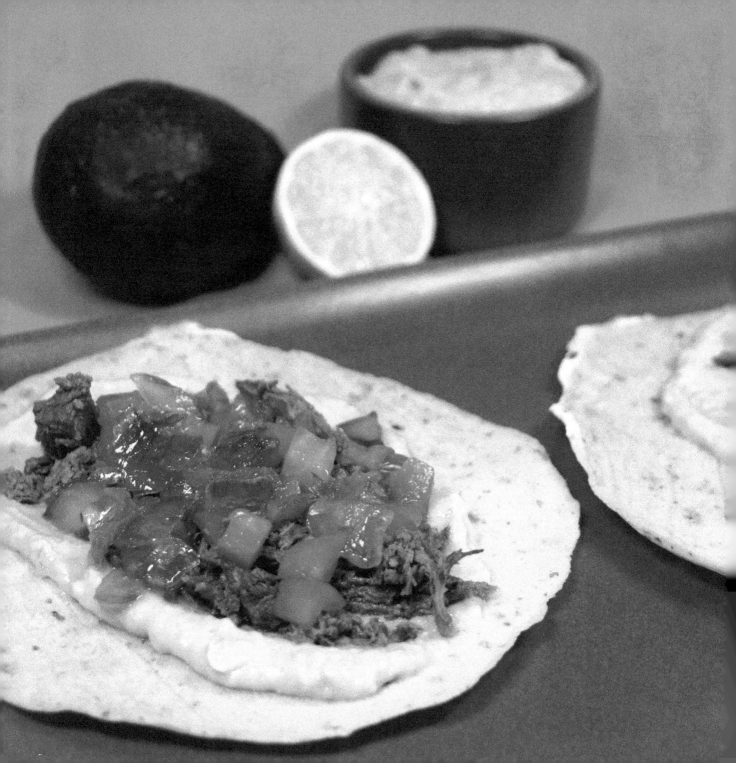

Tacos

Top 8 Free, Free From: Gluten, Cane Sugar, Coconut, Corn, Legumes, Mustard, Nightshades, Seeds, Sesame, Sulfites

Compatible With: AIP, Paleo, Low Histamine

Ingredients:

Sweet Onions:

6 ounces Organic Purple Onion, sliced

6 tsp YS Honey

1 - 2 tsp Safe Oil

1/2 tsp Sea Salt

Tortillas:

2 cups Millet Flour, superfine

1/2 cup Sorghum Flour, superfine

1.5 cup Safe Water

2 1/4 tsp Celtic Sea Salt

2 tsp Organic Dried Parsley

2 tsp Organic Onion Granules

1 tsp Organic Crushed Red Pepper

You'll Also Need:

Avocado Cream Sauce (page 39)

Shredded Bison (page 86)

Safe Tomatoes, diced

Directions:

For your onions, cut the root and stem off. Remove the skin, then slice in half. Slice each half into thin pieces. The final result is lots of "onion strings". Place your onion in a large pan with the olive oil, honey, and salt. Cook on medium-high heat for 10 minutes, stirring frequently.

For the tortillas, combine all of the ingredients together in a bowl. Follow the instructions for your tortilla press. We personally use parchment paper on our press, and cook our tortillas on the medium setting.

To assemble, spread avocado cream sauce on your tortillas and top with bison, sweet onions, and safe tomato.

For AIP: Use 2.5 cups Cassava instead of Millet and Sorghum. Omit tomatoes & crushed red pepper.

For Paleo: Use 2.5 cups Cassava instead of Millet and Sorghum.

For Low Histamine: Omit tomatoes.

Bacon Bomb Potatoes

Vegan, Top 8 Free, Free From: Gluten, Cane Sugar, Coconut, Corn, Legumes, Mustard, Seeds, Sesame, Sulfites

Friendly To: Low Histamine

These potatoes have become a staple in our home, as the kids simply adore them. This is an awesome meal to prepare before bed to make breakfast time a breeze.

Ingredients:

2 pounds Safe Potatoes, cubed

Safe Oil OR Bacon Lard (saved from cooking)

1 1/4 tsp Celtic Sea Salt

1 tsp Organic Smoked Paprika

3/4 tsp Organic Rosemary Powder

3 tsp Fresh Chopped Garlic

3 tsp Organic Onion Granules

1 TBSP Dried Organic Parsley

Other Seasoning Suggestions:

Salt, fresh chopped garlic, onion granules, parsley

Salt, smoked paprika, maple sugar

Salt, thyme, onion granules, black pepper

Directions:

There are so many ways to season your potatoes, which is great, because it helps prevent boredom. The technique to make these:

In a large mixing bowl, combine your cubed potatoes, oil of choice, and seasonings. You'll want to use enough oil or lard to coat the potatoes and prevent burning. When using lard, we use three large heaping spoons. Mix well. Transfer to a baking tray and bake at 425 for 20 minutes. The potatoes are done when they're easy to pierce with a fork.

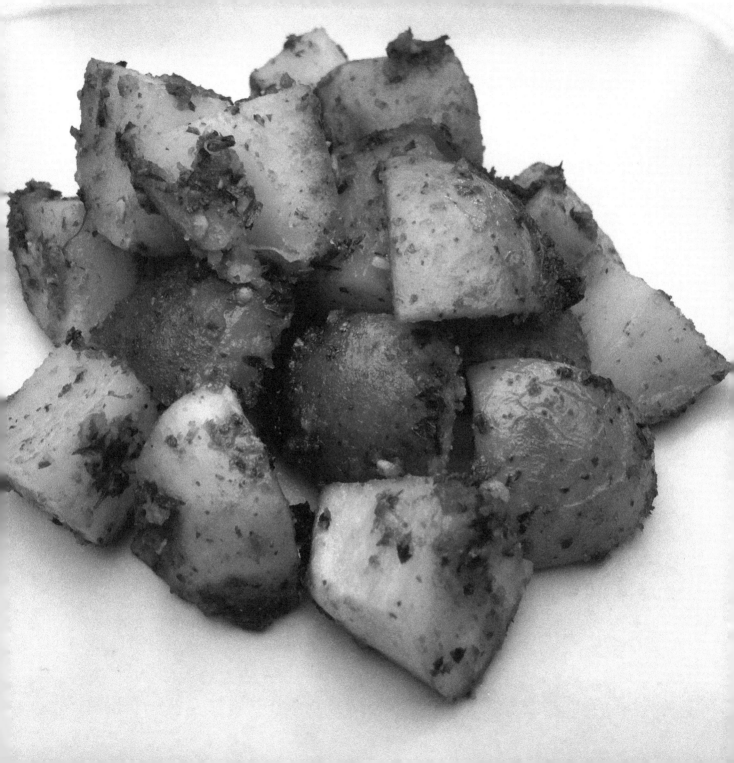

Inspiration Gallery

The recipes in this book only scratch the surface of what you can create safely. With the right basics, there are an infinite number of possibilities. Pictured: Grain Free Cookies, Chocolate Chia Pudding, Spicy Cupcakes, Sandwich Bread, Avocado Ice Cream, Fudgey Brownies with Caramel, Cinnamon Ginger Cake, and Freezer Pie.

All of these items were created without the top 8 allergens, gluten, legumes, or corn. Where do you go from here? Everywhere!! Sloppy Joe, pasta with cream sauce, homemade yogurt, frosting in so many flavors, cake, more waffles, cookies in too many flavors to count, and well, you get the idea. We're only limited by our imaginations. If you're looking for more ideas, be sure to connect with us online:

AllergyExpedition.com
A nationwide tour that brings resources and help directly to those that need it the most. The first annual tour was six weeks through 25 states, with more than 30 events.

FreeAndFriendlyFoods.com
A bakery in the San Francisco Bay Area. It's top 8 free, vegan, and much more. We have truly corn free options, Paleo, GAPs, AIP, and diabetic options as well.

FoodAndLego.com
This is our blog with hundreds of free recipes. There are all sorts of allergy needs being met, including onion, garlic, coconut, herbs, and everything in between.

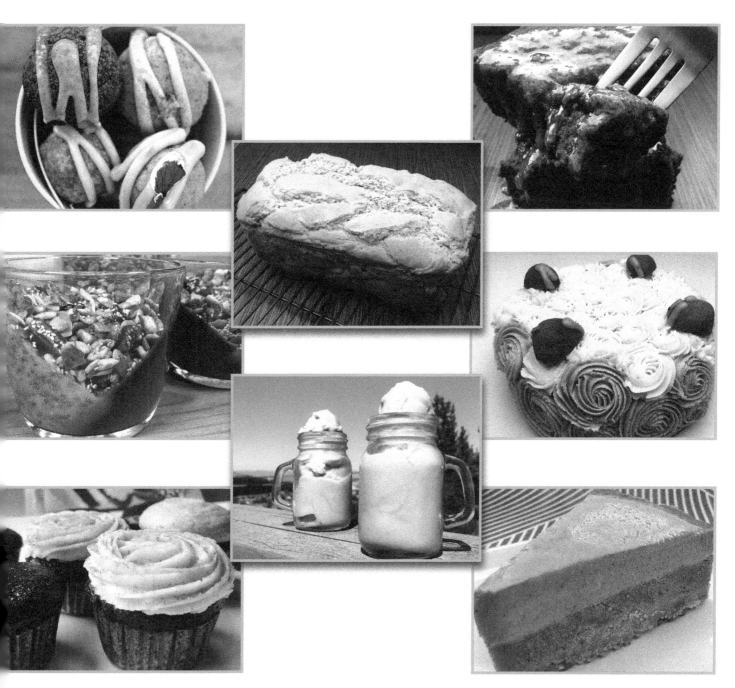